Better Than Before

How Overcoming Depression and Obesity Led to One Mom's Wellness Transformation

Emily Wright Mitchell

LEGACY launch pad PUBLISHING

ISBN [EBOOK]: 978-1-964377-84-1

ISBN [PAPERBACK]: 978-1-964377-86-5

To get Emily's 7-day reset, go to www.betterthanemily.com/reset
or scan the QR code below

CONTENTS

PART ONE

"Everything can be taken from a man but one thing: the last of human freedoms—to choose one's attitude in any given set of circumstances, to choose one's own way."

– Viktor Frankl

1 THE DARKNESS WAS ALL TOO CONSUMING

I LAID THERE STARING AT MY HUSBAND. I WAS GETTING READY TO tell him something big, something I wasn't sure if he'd be able to understand—that *I* didn't really understand myself. Up until that moment, I thought depression was a choice, or something that only happened to people with a lot of trauma or unfortunate circumstances. I didn't realize that when we don't heal past wounds or treat ourselves with the right words and actions—or when we just stop taking care of ourselves—it affects our health and can snowball into something we cannot ignore. This experience itself creates trauma.

When my depression became too consuming, I thought that I must have done something to cause it. I thought it was something I could control—or at least something that would resolve itself quickly if I listened to happy music, read a good book, took a hot shower or got more sleep. I thought that I could care for myself in the way that I do when I have a bad day, and that after a day or two, the depression would lift and I would feel normal again. But this was different.

I didn't know that hormones could affect your mental state—or that they could affect your entire life for extended periods of time. I didn't know that paranoia is something real, and that it hinders your ability to think clearly or even do basic problem-solving for yourself.

This time, the depression and anxiety weren't something I could shake, despite all the hot showers, positive reframing thoughts or active, hands-on help. The ground beneath me felt like shifting sand. It was getting so bad that I couldn't even attempt to control it. It was bigger than me. Earlier in the day, my husband had found me lying on the makeshift cot next to the crib, wearing pajamas covered in baby vomit.

Now it was 3:00 and I had been awake for most of the night. I hadn't slept for more than one hour at a time in days. As I would lay awake keeping my baby alive, I could feel anger rising in my body. I imagined that the rest of the world was fast asleep in the comfort of their beds. I believed that everyone on the planet was sleeping but me and this little baby who depended on me for survival. I needed to tell him how real this was for me. How this time, my depression and anxiety was unlike anything I'd ever experienced before.

"I can't do this anymore," I confessed, too weary and tired to be dramatic. "It's too much." I cried. "I've got to get some help."

I didn't even recognize my voice. I had lost all perspective and there was no plan helping to lift the dread that I was feeling. Even though my parents were helping out, I wasn't getting any sleep, and the feeling of isolation was growing in intensity. The fear and panic were also growing. The smallest of inconveniences, like the baby crying, felt insurmountable. It was like I had reached the edge of what I could handle as a human being. I had no ability to self-soothe. I couldn't imagine a world where I could say to myself *maybe everything is not that bad* or *what if everything works out?* I didn't see things in that way anymore, and I found myself unable to reframe my thoughts at all.

My husband was supportive and would do whatever it took to help me. He'd never seen me like this before, and I think it scared him a little. It scared me, too. I'd always been able to rebound before. I'd ask myself, *Why can't I just rebound this time?* while feeling like I was doing something wrong. I had come out of bad times or feelings of anxiety in the past without having to ask for help or get anyone else involved with my inner thoughts.

I didn't believe that depression could happen to someone like me. I had support, stability and a caring community. Wasn't I supposed to just nap this off? Didn't I just have a bout of "baby blues" like other moms I knew?

Or was it something worse? I wondered all the time, *if this is something worse, how in the world will I have the time to figure this out? I barely have time now. I can't even take a shower and blow-dry my hair without the baby crying and needing me for soothing.* But that's the funny thing about time and how you spend it. When you reach rock bottom—whether it's a terrifying diagnosis or a life-altering event—the only thing you have time for is damage control. This wasn't going away without effort. I could either spend my time spiraling more and more out of control, or healing. It was up to me.

How bad is too bad? That was the question I kept asking myself. *When is the right time to let people in on how dark my thoughts had become?* I didn't know. I was ashamed of my feelings. Ashamed of how disconnected I was from my babies, how I didn't feel I was bonding with my son, how I hadn't had a positive feeling in weeks. I was terrified of telling the truth. Terrified that they might deem me unfit, a failure.

When I looked in the mirror, I was unrecognizable. Staring back at me was someone who had doubled in size, someone who didn't move her body and depended on food to cope with feelings of fear and shame. Being thin was the ultimate goal for most of my life. How had I let this happen? Seeing myself this way was the physical evidence that things had gotten out of control. My inability to fix it made me dislike myself. This inability to feel anything, to take action, was the hardest part. I was stuck and I had no idea how to get out.

I tried telling other moms I knew about the struggles I was

having. I would tell them that the exhaustion was making it hard for me to function and that I wasn't feeling any joy. "I'm just so tired, you know?" I found myself telling another mom one day. I hoped that she would follow up with how hard things had been for her and share in this pain with me. "Have you tried sleeping when the baby sleeps?" she asked me.

"Yeah, I know, I need to get better about doing that," I said, feeling completely let down and even more isolated. Maybe though, this other mom felt reluctant to share her pain out of fear and paranoia, just like me. It's possible that she felt isolated, too.

Of course, we can only process our thoughts at the level that we have awareness about what is happening around us. When you become a mom, every single thing about your life changes overnight. Each new mother now has a responsibility to care for her unique baby's needs with whatever tools and knowledge they have. They are learning to care for their new baby and figuring out their own needs while recovering from childbirth, which is hard on a woman's body. The body undergoes such dramatic changes that everything—from the way you process emotions to how you digest your food—is completely out of whack. All the things that used to work no longer help. Everything you used to know is gone and you must relearn a new way.

In those early years of parenting, many of my mom friends didn't have any idea what was truly happening in their bodies and how to function in their new roles. We all did the very best that we could with the information that we had access to at that time. I could have never known what another woman was going through behind closed doors.

But now I was growing paranoid. When my parents came over to help out, I could hear them in the other room, whispering about me with my husband. I lacked the energy or confidence to interrupt them and tell them I was fine. I just let them whisper about me in my own home while I sat on the couch mentally unable to do anything about it. Part of me hoped that while they were whispering, they would come up with an answer. I hoped that they would come back into the room and tell me that they had figured it all out and now everything could go back to normal. They didn't have the answers. They all knew that something was off, that this wasn't me, but we lacked the resources or the understanding of what to do. I felt like I was becoming a statistic that you hear about on the nightly news. It was like an out-of-body experience. While I now know it's one that so many women face, at the time, I felt like I must be the only one.

Postpartum depression is a type of depression that occurs during pregnancy or in the first year after giving birth. PPD is the most common complication for women who have just had a baby. It's estimated that about 1 in 7 women are at risk for developing PPD. For half of the women who are diagnosed with PPD, it is their first experience with major depression. This was true for me. Although I'd struggled with a low level of anxiety and depression in the past, this was completely foreign to me.

The Mayo Clinic says that there is no one cause for PPD, but that there are many factors that can play a role in determining whether or not someone will develop it[i]. One contributing factor is physical changes in the body.

After childbirth, the body goes through a drastic disruption of hormones such as progesterone and estrogen. These fluctuations in hormones can be another major factor in determining whether or not someone might develop PPD. I always refer to childbirth as a rocket launch for moms. When the baby comes out, everything else gets destroyed on the way out. Your body goes through physical and hormonal changes, and many of these changes can affect your mood.

During the time of my pregnancies, postpartum depression was becoming more common. In fact, research shows that postpartum depression rates are increasing every year. This could be because more women are feeling comfortable sharing about their experiences or because more women's studies are reported. I think it's probably both. The more we learn that these struggles are a part of a shared experience, the more we feel comfortable talking about it to each other and seeking help from medical care providers.

Even though PPD wasn't something I knew much about, I'd spent my whole life gearing up for it. I had no idea that the habits I formed as an adolescent—my years of yo-yo dieting, lack of movement during pregnancy and dependence on food as a coping mechanism—were likely increasing my symptoms. Some studies have shown that a diet of refined grains, sugary treats and processed foods—along with low intakes of fruits and vegetables—is associated with an increased risk of depression. During this time, those were about the only foods that I was eating—processed junk food with no nutritional value at all.

In the book *Good Energy,* author Casey Means says that sometimes we have to look upstream and question why the symptoms are there. She encourages women to ask questions when they're in doubt about what is happening in their brains and bodies. She says to ask yourself, *Could inflammation due to an unhealthy lifestyle cause psychological distress?* The answer to this is usually yes. And in my case, it was definitely yes. But at this time, my symptoms were already so out of control that this basic logic was not accessible to me.

When my doctor diagnosed me with PPD and explained that my symptoms would persist without some kind of intervention, my logic finally kicked back in. Hearing her say that it would not get better on its own made something click inside me. I thought about the things I had done to help myself and came up empty. I was too deep in my depression to even think about interventions. Seeing my doctor and hearing that I would have to help myself was a turning point. I suddenly woke up to my life and began to wonder what things I could try at home to reduce my symptoms. *Maybe there are some things I can do about this,* I thought. *Maybe there is hope.*

In *Good Energy,* Means goes on to say that it's not currently part of the medical culture to ask questions about the symptoms that we are experiencing. Something about my interaction with my doctor that day reminded me of this. Even though I was in the darkest place I'd ever been emotionally, I still had a deep curiosity and was ready to ask myself the questions that needed to be asked, even if no one else was. There was a deep knowing within me that the only way that I was going to heal was if I changed.

Still, change itself is a stressful event, even if it leads to positive outcomes. I had reached such a low point that I would do anything if it might lead to relief. I remember telling my mom once, "If there was a 12-step program for this, I would do it." To me, doing a program like the 12-Steps (which is the primary course of treatment in Alcoholics Anonymous and is designed to help you recover from alcohol addiction) made sense. You follow this plan, there's a group of people who help hold you accountable and support you when you need help and, following the plan, you begin to heal.

The funny thing about mental and emotional trauma is that there is no step-by-step process, and there is no set time for when you will heal. I felt like I was staring at an overgrown grass field, stretching taller than I could stand. I didn't have a riding lawn mower, just someone handing me a weed whacker as if to say, *let's move forward slowly and see what we find as we go.* I wasn't used to this. In the past, every time I wanted something, I was able to white-knuckle my way through. This was going to be different. I could already see that there was no quick fix.

Even though I was ready for change, I'm still shocked by what I was able to understand in that moment of desperation. Challenging how you see life can be really overwhelming, but I had no choice than to try. My babies needed a mother and I had to take care of myself. I had a deep inner knowledge that this was my responsibility. Now the question I needed to ask myself was, to paraphrase Viktor Frankl, *how would I choose my last freedom in all of these circumstances?* I had to both discover an attitude that allowed me to thrive and figure out how I would find that attitude. I knew that nothing was going to change here but me. I asked myself how I would answer this call.

2 HOW IT ALL BEGAN: GROWING UP IN THE '90S

I GREW UP IN A COASTAL TOWN JUST 15 MINUTES FROM THE BEACH IN Corpus Christi, Texas. It was a small community where everyone knew everyone's name. I spent my childhood in a place where people were always happy to see each other and where I felt welcome no matter what. When I was little my parents, brother and I would spend our entire weekends at the beach. I loved playing in the sand dunes and building sandcastles. We would spend the day swimming and fishing, and even trying to surf. At the end of a beach day like this I felt completely fulfilled and tired from the waves knocking me down over and over again. I felt connected to my parents and my brother as we laughed each time the surf board would slip away.

There was a freedom about these days together. This was back when I could be on the beach in my swimsuit and *not* think about my body. I would run around on the hot sand, unconcerned with what I looked like, if my swimsuit was right for my body shape or what others might think of me. I was free, free from the chatter of my mind. I wasn't comparing myself to others or sizing myself up to other girls my age. These were the days that my mind was present on what I was doing at the moment. It was a time of pure childhood innocence.

My childhood home was in a middle-class neighborhood lined with three-bedroom, two-bath ranches. My parents were both teachers, working on their Master of Education degrees. My mom had hopes of becoming an elementary school principal, which she later accomplished. My parents put in long hours as teachers. My dad often stayed after school to coach sports. When they were finished with their day jobs they took classes in order to earn their advanced degrees. They raised my brother and I, instilling important family values. Our needs were always met and we never felt like my parents were working any harder than anyone else we knew. I know it wasn't always easy, but they never let my brother and I in on any struggles that they were having at that time.

When my dad was younger, he was an All-American football player. He's in the Liberty University Hall of Fame for defensive line. He is 6'3, has red hair and is stronger than anyone I know. When I was little, I was in awe of his strength and his ability to easily pick up and excel at any sport. He carried his love for football and teamwork into adulthood and became a football coach at my school.

But my dad's heart was bigger than his physical strength. As a coach he had a profound impact on the kids that he worked with in our community. He had a leadership style that really taught others how to take care of each other. He showed me how to be a leader and had a servant leadership style, always putting others first. He focused on decisions for the greater good not just for the team, but for humanity.

Once, when I was little, I got caught lying. My dad lectured me on the importance of having integrity. I'll never forget asking him what integrity meant and why I should care about it. My dad explained who we are on the inside, saying that integrity holds us together and makes us healthy. He stressed how important it is to live as our authentic selves, that we are who we say we are. He explained that loving other people and supporting them is more important than winning or having selfish pleasures that don't serve the greater good. I understood then that lying wasn't worth hurting someone else. While that lesson didn't greatly impact me at the moment, it was something that I come back to through my struggles. He planted a seed that authenticity was important.

From the time I started school until around age 10, my brother and I stayed with my dad every day after school. My mom was in school in the evenings, and my dad coached most after-school sports. When he wasn't coaching, he ran the weight room at school. It was open for all athletes to come and lift. We loved staying with him at the gym. When the bell rang, we would head straight to the gym where my dad was finishing up his classes and getting ready to coach his players. Sometimes, after his last class and before his first player would arrive, he would squeeze in a weight lifting session for himself or play with us at the gym. Usually we would play H-O-R-S-E or organize a basketball game with whoever was available. We were active and he was leading us.

During the summer months, we would still go to the gym with our dad. At first, I would just play on the weight machines alongside my dad, not really knowing how they worked. My dad also taught us how to lift weights. I would try to lift the heavy bar with my little brother spotting me, or I would sit on the leg machine and push the heavy weights up and down with all my might. I'll never forget this one time when my dad was teaching me to lift the bar. He would roll up this towel and put it right between my chest bones to protect my chest. I think he was afraid that lifting would stunt my growth because I was a female. This still makes me laugh. I'm grateful that he was teaching me about strength building at such a young age. He was showing me to value physical fitness, which I did for many years.

My dad encouraged me to play sports. Being in the gym my entire childhood helped me become a decent athlete. I could pick up on how to play sports quickly and loved basketball, volleyball, softball and running. My dad loved to watch me play sports and even though his job was coaching, he never tried to coach me during my games. He never wanted to pressure me. He knew how much I loved to play sports and really liked watching me play. Unlike other things in my life, sports felt natural and easy. It allowed me to feel part of a community. It was a built-in structure for movement and activity which I now know directly affected my mental health. I learned how to make decisions for the greater good of the team, push my body to learn and grow stronger and to support something I cared about no matter if we won or lost.

In addition to an active lifestyle, our family dinners were also an important value when I was growing up. Almost every night, at dinnertime, my parents turned off the TV and engaged my brother and I in discussion about the highs and lows of our day. My mom made recipes that came off the back of Campbell's soup cans. Enchilada casserole, king chicken casserole, taco casserole and Hamburger Helper were our dinnertime staples, just like most of America. This was the food everyone was eating.

While my family had a strong background in physical fitness, when it came to nutrition, we lacked knowledge. When I wasn't eating home-cooked meals, I ate packaged foods, freezer meals and fast food—often. With our busy schedules, fast food became a new constant. Fast food was a solution for most families (and still is today). It's much easier to manage dinner time when everyone is going a million directions and eating at all different times based on their different schedules.

As I got older and had more choice over what I would eat, I found that I *always* chose fast food. Some days, I would eat McDonald's for breakfast, Taco Bell for lunch and pizza dipped in ranch dressing for dinner. To say I wasn't getting the necessary nutrients I needed from food is an understatement. It's not that packaged foods or pizza dipped in ranch (my favorite) are *bad,* but they became problematic when they were the only foods I consumed.

There was a deeper reason I was so drawn to processed foods. Do you remember slogans like "once you pop you can't stop"? During the '80s, processed food companies (like Kraft and Nabisco) were bought by Phillip Morris (you know him as the founder of Big Tobacco) and soon their employees began working on developing something called a "bliss point." According to a 2023 *Washington Post* article, "the term *bliss point* had emerged as a crucial concept in understanding the sales success of any particular heavily processed product." The "bliss point" refers to the perfect balance of sugar, salt and fat that makes a food item irresistible. In essence, this means that they were creating nutrient-poor products that can take over the brain's reward system, leading to cravings and compulsive eating behaviors. These food companies' whole focus was quite literally (and still is) to get us hooked so we consume more of their product.

So, it wasn't just that I had no nutritional guidance; my brain was being altered by the processed foods I was eating. I was craving more and more unhealthy foods and had less desire to eat foods like protein, which would have left me feeling satiated without the additional chemical reactions in my brain. Not only had my brain's reward system been groomed, I struggled with acne, low mood, low energy and inflammation.

As I got older I began to gain weight. Not only were my hormones shifting, but also the food I was eating was affecting my hormones. It was a pivotal time in my life as an adolescent girl and it felt like I had changed overnight. *What in the world is wrong with me?* I thought, feeling puffy and bloated. This was when I began to develop negotiating skills. I figured out that if I cut back on some foods, that I might not gain as much weight. So I would plan to restrict myself a bit, telling myself I would feel better if I just ate a Nestle Crunch ice cream bar for lunch and no pizza. I was totally clueless as to how to restrict my diet, but I was learning that restriction might actually work.

I didn't know how to manage food in a healthy way. It never occurred to me that the way I was eating could affect my mood. I had no idea that organic meat and fresh vegetables could go a long way in helping me meet my nutritional needs. And even if I had, this type of eating wasn't popular or accessible. No one in my life knew what organic food was, and even if they had, there weren't many options for finding this kind of food.

Who could blame my parents for feeding me convenience and prepackaged foods? They were both working full time and going to school. Foods that were packaged, canned or boxed meant that we could still sit down to eat together as a family but no one had to spend hours in the kitchen. This was what the American people were asking for—foods that would fit into the new busy lifestyles of working families. Most people saw this as a win and wouldn't know the true outcomes for many years. People rarely thought of food as a product to be marketed—and that some of the advertising claims about nutritional content just weren't true.

In junior high, I hit puberty and my body began to change. I was gaining weight and felt bloated a lot of the time. My clothes felt tight and I began to feel uncomfortable. I began to wonder why I couldn't seem to effortlessly look the way I wanted to look. I didn't feel like I looked like other girls in junior high. I remember once at school, we were required to do a physical fitness test in P.E. To complete the exam, I had to stand on a scale and weigh myself while a teacher recorded it on the clipboard. I stood in line nervously, waiting for my turn. When I was next, I stood on the scale and saw what I feared was a heavy weight for my age and height. I watched my teacher record my weight at 147 pounds. As she wrote down the number next to my name, I scanned the sheet to look at everyone else's weight. I saw 120 pounds, 122 pounds, and even 125 pounds. My worst nightmare was true. I weighed more than all the other kids in my class.

After the test, I saw a group of girls gathered in the corner talking about their weight. They all weighed about the same yet were still comparing the differences of just one or two pounds. One of the girls approached me.

"How much do you weigh, Emily?" she asked. I began to panic, and I didn't know what to tell her. I knew my weight was more than every other girl there, but I just couldn't bring myself to say the number—which to me at this point seemed astronomical—out loud. "I weigh 125," I lied, abandoning the lesson that my dad taught me about being my true authentic self. As soon as I said it, I knew it was a mistake. One girl in particular doubted me. I could feel my heart banging in my chest. I felt vulnerable and afraid. I had a gut feeling that she knew the truth.

Later, I discovered she did find out my true weight. She looked at it on the clipboard after we had all walked away, then spread the news to all the girls in my class. I regretted lying; I was mortified. It was right then and there I hated my body. This was the beginning of me despising who I was solely based on my comparison to others. I felt like I needed to be more *like them* and less like myself.

This wasn't my only realization that I was different. Around this same time, I noticed that my mom started making comments on the clothes that I wore. I felt like she had high expectations of my brother and me. We were always expected to look our best at all times, keep our rooms clean and use our manners. But suddenly I felt like she was putting a lot of focus on my body, too. Looking back, I realize that she was trying to protect me the best way she knew how. She wanted to make sure that as I started to gain weight, I still presented myself well and kept my clothes looking appropriate. However, in my 13-year-old mind, all I heard when she commented on my clothes was that *you are different, you will never be where you want to be.* I started to believe these lies that I told myself and my feelings of self hatred began to snowball.

Once in 8th grade, my mom and I went swimsuit shopping

with some friends. My friends had each picked out a cute bikini to try on and I chose one too, which I felt pretty good about wearing. When we all came out I was excited to see how I looked until I heard my mom talking with my friends.

"Emily's body isn't made for a two-piece swimsuit. Emily is more fitted for a one-piece or a tankini that covers her stomach completely." I felt crushed. *What was wrong with my body?* I thought. *Is my body so bad that people would be offended if they saw it?*

"Mom, please!" I begged, trying to convince her that my body was good enough to wear a bikini. But there was no arguing with her, she wouldn't have it any other way.

I looked at my friends, feeling humiliated. Here I was again, so badly wanting to wear what they were wearing and look like them, with thin bodies that seemed normal.

This incident was an intense source of shame and the beginning of what would be a very unhealthy relationship with how I felt about my body. I coped by desperately trying to shrink; it was a physical manifestation of my emotional state. I would stand in a manner that said *just let me be invisible.* I would hunch my shoulders, stand behind people, out of sight, trying to be still and quiet. If I was sitting on a couch, I would grab a pillow and put it on my lap to cover my stomach. *Just hide, cover up, don't allow yourself to be seen.*

I was good at running and liked being on the track, but that wasn't the real reason I ran. I decided to join the track team because I thought running would be good for weight loss, and it was. My dad ran every morning before work and he encouraged me to run with him. He believed that I got up at 5 am to run with him so that I could meet goals of getting faster and being able to compete. I was just doing it to lose weight. Once during our morning run, I mentioned to my dad that I felt like I was struggling to keep weight off like other girls.

"Dad, I just can't seem to be thin, no matter how much I run. Maybe it's the food we eat?" I asked. "I mean, I do eat a lot of fast food, and I love to eat pizza dipped in ranch." My dad listened to me, but he didn't make the connection between my size and the food I was eating. So, at the time, neither did I.

While nutrition wasn't an important topic at the time, dieting was. I remember heavily marketed restriction diets like the *Special K* diet, which at the time was described as being balanced and healthy. On the *Special K* diet you eat a bowl of cereal for breakfast, a bowl for lunch and then have a light dinner. This wasn't the only diet like this. *Slim Fast* was also insanely popular at this time, and it had the same concept: a shake for breakfast, a shake for lunch and then a light dinner. These companies weren't as interested in creating healthy communities. They were interested in making sales. If you did the *Special K* diet, you were going to need to buy a lot of cereal. And if two of your meals each day were replaced by a certain brand of shakes, you would need to buy a lot of those, too.

We consumers all took these ideas at face value. At the time, we believed that these companies had information that they wanted to share—and we bought into it without questioning the motives behind the claims. These diets *did* work. I remember seeing people lose weight using these methods of restriction—but losing weight didn't necessarily mean being healthy. These meal replacements lacked the essential nutrients and proteins that our bodies need to function optimally. Regardless, I watched the adults around me hop onto these yo-yo diets in hopes that they would see the promised results. They had no knowledge or information about the other issues this kind of dieting can create.

It is only now that I can understand how harmful these dieting tactics are, and that is only because I've increased my knowledge of nutrition through extensive research. The truth of what was happening was out there, but it was really hard to find. It takes time and effort to discover the truth about dieting, marketing and nutrition. Most people want a quicker fix. When it comes to nutrition, we must get to a place where we question information and find out for ourselves what is accurate.

Beyond the "bliss point," food company executives were learning new ways to market and sell food, creating the booming business of dieting. A *Forbes* article from 2021 called "Dieting For Dollars: How Food & Beverage Companies Can Fatten the Bottomline" shows how food businesses have created big opportunities out of marketing diets to consumers. It reports that about 45 million Americans start a diet each year, spending $33 billion annually on weight loss products.

I was learning about nutrition at the same time food companies were ramping up this marketing to sell more food. My foundation for food choices was established right alongside the food pyramid which was developed in 1992 by the United States Department Of Agriculture (USDA) as an educational tool for Americans. Almost as soon as it was developed and released, medical professionals and other experts questioned its validity. Some critics even said that it was responsible for contributing to the obesity crisis[i]. But it was too late: the food pyramid was already posted in our school cafeterias, on the back of our cereal boxes and printed in our textbooks. Most people believed that eating six servings of grains and limiting protein was good for you. And by grains, many people took that to mean sugary cereals, white bread, pasta and rice.

According to some doctors and nutritionists, the food pyramid was based on outdated, inaccurate information. It recommended up to 11 servings of bread, cereal, rice and pasta daily, and it suggested 2-3 servings each of meat and dairy without specifying lean or low-fat sources. Fats were generally to be avoided. "Because of the bread and grain focus, even if you ate within calorie limits, you still missed out on the vitamins, minerals and fiber you needed to stay healthy," says UAB Medicine Diabetes and Nutrition Education Clinic Supervisor Barbara Roberts, MS, RDN, LDN, CDE. "The pyramid didn't recommend *whole* grains specifically, which help combat type 2 diabetes."[ii] The food pyramid was later amended in 2005 and again in 2011 to something called My Plate.

Today, there are studies that show that eating processed foods can lead to physical issues. If you're mainly eating processed foods, it's more likely that you are not consuming other foods like fruits and vegetables. Fruits and vegetables have essential nutrients that your brain needs in order to function optimally. Without these vital nutrients, you're at risk for developing chronic physical health issues.

In addition to physical health issues, many studies[iii] have shown that because adolescence is such a critical period for psychological changes, eating a diet high in ultra-processed foods can lead to depression.

Without this information, my poor eating habits were taking a toll on both my brain and my body. By eighth grade, I was addicted to processed foods, I hated the way my body looked and I was beginning to have feelings of isolation. I believed I was the anomaly in the family—the *one* person who didn't have it together when it came being the right size. No matter how hard I worked out or exercised, the weight just wouldn't budge. I couldn't meet the impossible standards that I felt were expected of me. I knew I was letting everyone down, including myself. I needed to do something about this, and soon I would find a solution.

3 CRACK THIN IS IN

BY THE TIME I HIT HIGH SCHOOL, I HAD ADOPTED THE IDEA THAT NO matter how hard I worked to lose weight, I was just "big boned." How could I not come to this conclusion? I had tried as many different kinds of strategies for weight loss as possible while working out as much as I could, and yet nothing seemed to move the needle like I hoped. My weight was still higher than I wanted it to be. Sure, I had some success, but it never lasted for longer than a few weeks. I began to wonder if it was a faulty genetic makeup that I would just have to live with. I started to believe that since I was "big boned," there was no chance for me to obtain the results I so badly wanted. I wondered, *are my bones actually bigger than other peoples'?* As a result, I decided that my problem must be genetics.

When I flipped through magazines or saw girls on TV, they were all thin. I wanted to look like them. This was the time when thinness was glamorized, and models like Kate Moss were praised for their bodies. This was also the era of MTV. MTV went live for spring break, where they showed bands playing of course, but more importantly, girls dancing in their swimsuits. There seemed to be a massive media presence perpetuating ideas of what young women should look like (particularly in bathing suits). Every girl I saw on TV seemed to be a carbon copy of exactly what I wanted to look like; a tall, thin girl, with a beautiful face and great hair. When I saw these girls on TV, I believed their lives must be full of fun and happiness, that they must be content and proud of their bodies. This look and lifestyle became my ultimate goal, and I was ready to do whatever it took to reach it.

One day at school I overheard a girl I was jealous of talking with some friends. She was a cheerleader and came across as very confident. She seemed happy, had a lot of friends around her at all times, and, most importantly, she was thin. She was talking about her body and mentioned her diet plan.

"How does your body look so good?" her friend asked her.

"Oh, it's my diet," she replied. "I just don't eat very much."

"What do you eat?" her friend asked.

"Oh, like one candy bar a day," she giggled and then walked away, taking her perfect skinny body with her.

That's what I'm going to do, I thought to myself and almost immediately my new diet was underway. I was going to starve myself.

I started on a new diet that consisted of diet pills, one Snapple and one slice of bread. I also used laxatives "as necessary" to get the water weight off. I could easily buy everything I needed for my new diet in one quick trip to the drug store. At this time, diet pills were popular and everyone took them, including my mom. I had no reason to believe that they were anything but safe. I wasn't sure exactly how they worked, but I knew that when I took them, I didn't feel hungry. I washed them down with my Snapple and ate my slice of bread as if it were the most normal thing in the world. As a highschooler, the cost of this kind of dieting didn't matter to me. All I cared about was looking thin, and I was aiming to see the quickest results. I wasn't alone either–this was a popular strategy for a lot of young women my age.

Diet pills are appetite suppressants that block certain brain chemicals. These medications were studied for their great effectiveness for weight loss. At the time they were released however, there were no long-term studies done on how they might impact the brain and body. No one cared. Millions of Americans used these pills without fear. They were the solution that many women longed for, a quick and easy weight loss approach that worked!

Later, many diet pills were taken off the market for their connection to heart issues. But by that time, I was already using them regularly and seeing the weight loss results I was seeking. I didn't have the maturity or the skills to weigh the costs of using diet pills as a tool for weight loss. And even if I had, I'm not sure that I would have stopped. It was the first time that I was seeing results. I was finally thin.

My use of laxatives as a tool for weight loss was also quite unsafe. Overuse of laxatives can block nutrient absorption and increase intestinal issues. Laxatives were a quick fix. They helped me get the water weight off in order to look good for a party or a school function. My stomach felt flat and therefore I had relief, albeit brief, from hating my body.

My methods were working. The weight started melting off, and soon I was being praised for my new look. Friends at school and even adults would approach me and compliment me on my "hard work." I heard compliments like, *"You're so small!"*, *"You have such amazing discipline!"* and *"You're so motivated!"* They all reinforced the idea that starving myself was a successful strategy. I felt proud of my accomplishments.

My body was thinning. It was exactly what I thought I needed to feel happy and less anxious. But my body hatred wasn't lifting, even with my new size. I started to resent the fact that I had to starve myself to look thin. I believed that other skinny people were born that way and that they didn't have to work at it. I was frustrated. Even though I was getting complimented on my new look, in my mind, I still looked like I did before. I couldn't see the person staring back at me in the mirror. Instead, I saw my middle school self—bloated and husky.

I was sucked into a vortex; constantly chasing success, never feeling like I was ever enough. No amount of weight loss led to any kind of happiness. Despite this, I continued to chase happiness by dieting and restricting food. It would be years before I understood that it's impossible to become happier by just looking a certain way. At the time, I believed that my life would get better on the other side of my perceived appearance issues. I couldn't see or love myself while I was in that kind of mental state. As long as I continued down that path, I was never going to be enough. And all the while, I was treating my body poorly and with contempt, mirroring how I felt about myself.

At school, I still felt really insecure in my body. I never felt like my clothes fit right and I was becoming obsessed with comparing myself to other girls my age. I remember one homecoming football game. I was feeling insecure as usual, and tried my best to make myself small enough to not be noticed. I was standing with a small group of girls when some cheerleaders ran over.

"Come on!" one of them said, while grabbing the hands of the girls standing around me.

"Let's all get out on the field and cheer on the team!" another cheerleader encouraged.

The girls I was standing with gladly ran along with the cheerleaders, excited to get a chance to be out on the field in front of the crowd.

I held back. There was no way that I could stand in front of anyone, let alone the whole school. I worried that my stomach was too flabby and that my shorts didn't look right. I wanted to hide my body away from everyone. I felt panicked on the inside. The mental chatter in my mind was going a mile a minute at that moment, saying things like *what if they can see that I'm breaking out? My smile is funny looking. I'm gonna look weird because I feel weird.* And finally, the one question that was always present: *Why can't I just be normal?*

Thinking about my body consumed me. My insecurity was growing. No matter where I was or what I was doing, I compared myself to the people around me. I would watch girls eat bags of chips and continue to maintain beautiful thin frames. Meanwhile, if I so much as sniffed Cheeto dust, I felt I was going to gain ten pounds. I was so angry about my "bad genes" that made me "big boned." I thought that things would never feel easy for me. I lived in a gigantic pity party with no way to self soothe and gain perspective.

Looking back, I realize that I had body dysmorphia, a distorted body image. A *Medical News Today* article calls it an obsessive and excessive preoccupation with a perceived physical flaw. A person with body dysmorphia may fixate on this perceived flaw to a degree that disrupts their life. This was exactly what I was experiencing at the time. I had begun to obsess about how my body looked and felt a compulsion to fix my appearance by getting thin. This compulsion was disruptive to my everyday life. There was nothing I could have done to make me feel good about myself. To me, my body was *wrong*, even if it looked fine to everyone else. I always felt too big despite my frame growing smaller and smaller. I felt like an imposter, a husky girl living in a skinny body.

I suspect that my body dysmorphia didn't come directly from low self-esteem; it can also develop because of a chemical imbalance in the brain. My restrictive diet was likely having an impact on my brain because I wasn't getting the nutrients that my brain needed to function optimally. In addition, I was at an age when my brain was still developing. In order for the brain to properly develop, it needs vitamins, which mostly come from food. Things like protein, whole grains and fruits and vegetables are essential foods for the teenage brain to develop. I wasn't getting any of those much needed vitamins and minerals.

While my mental health was starting to suffer, my diet

strategy wasn't impacting my athletic ability. My performance was still at its peak. One time, during softball practice, I had to run a mile. I ran it at a seven minute pace even though I'd barely eaten anything for days.

"How did you run that so fast?" my teammates asked me, knowing that I starved myself.

I wasn't sure. I could perform well even when I was so undernourished. I just thought of it as confirmation that starvation wasn't really so bad after all. When you're determined to reach your goals, there truly is nothing that will stop you. I was so determined during this time of my life. I thought things like *look how motivated I am, look how disciplined I am, I must be doing something right*. I felt like nothing else mattered as long as I got what I wanted: to be thin, to perform at my best and to have people compliment me on my hard work and discipline. Perfection was my goal. As long as I kept up this pace, I *was* perfect. I had to keep going.

Soon though, I started to experience serious consequences. My athletic life, the one place where I felt free from body obsession, was starting to cause me severe anxiety. I noticed that I was suddenly super anxious before games that used to be no big deal. I would feel extreme pressure to perform well and worry that if I didn't, I would let others down. I began to have thoughts like *there is something seriously wrong with me* and *why can't I just be normal?* I was already so ashamed of my body and suddenly it felt like I wasn't worthy enough to be anywhere, even at my own sporting events. The anxiety felt like one more thing I was doing wrong.

I started throwing up before my volleyball games. One night right before the game started, I ran into the bathroom and threw up. Before I ran back out to join the team I sat on my knees hovering over the toilet thinking to myself *why can't you get it together Emily? Normal people don't do this. You can't ever be normal.* I hid this from everyone. I couldn't stand the thought of anyone knowing how messed up I was becoming.

On the outside, I was being complimented and praised for my body. On the inside, no one knew the real toll that it was taking. I never tried hiding my dieting tactics. No one did. At the time, it wasn't taboo to talk about wanting to be skinny. All the girls at my school seemed to be on some kind of diet, like the cheerleader who only ate a candy bar a day, or other girls who also took diet pills or obsessively worked out. We all openly professed that it was only to lose weight. I, too, was vocal about what I ate and the fact that I took diet pills. All anyone seemed to care about was whether or not I was skinny.

One afternoon, I was walking home from school and one of my friends approached me. "Emily, you've lost a lot of weight," she said, with a concerned look on her face. "I notice that you don't eat much of anything at all."

I brushed it off, saying "Oh yeah! I've been taking diet pills in the morning and I'm not that hungry, so I just drink a Snapple and eat a piece of bread in the afternoon and that keeps me full."

I waited for the praise I had grown used to.

"Emily, that's really not good for you!" she said instead. "If you continue this and don't start eating more, I might have to get your mom involved."

I was too deep in my own self hatred to notice that what I was doing was unhealthy. Nothing mattered more than being thin. I looked at my friend and thought, *Who are you to judge me? Who are you to tell me what to do? You don't know what this is like to have to constantly starve to be thin!*

I'd finally gotten my weight under control and I was terrified of going backwards. I wasn't going to let this friend ruin it all for me. I decided right then and there that I would start hiding the truth. I wouldn't let people know how little I was eating or that I was taking diet pills and laxatives. This put a gap in our friendship. So much of my life was consumed with dieting and the desire to be thin, and I found that when I started hiding those things about myself, I hid a lot of other things too. This included my mental health struggles. We started to grow apart, mostly because I was now hiding my true self from her.

Over time, hiding myself started to cause a lot of guilt and shame. Even though I was still seeing the results that I wanted, my friend's comment lingered in the back of my mind. Here I was again, having to take extreme measures just to be normal like everyone else. The tactics that I had to use to get myself thin were taking a toll. My mental health began to suffer, but I still had no idea that it was diet-related.

What I know now is that not getting proper nourishment can affect your mental health as well as your physical health. Lacking the proper vitamins and proteins affects everything from your gut health to your brain. It can cause stress to the body at a cellular level. As cells become endangered, the whole body focuses on cell repair, which disrupts other natural systems. This affects your sleep and can even cause autoimmune disorders. When you're not fueling your body properly, the stress on your body is harsh and damaging.

In my effort to be thin, I was sacrificing all of the things that mattered when it came to my health. I was doing things that disrupted my bodily functions, likely making things harder for myself. Because I was still so young, I was able to manage like this for a while without having to face serious health consequences. I didn't develop an autoimmune issue or get sick more often, but this kind of living has a way of catching up to you. The younger you are, the more resilient you are, even to bad habits or a dangerous lifestyle. In my case, it didn't mean I was immune to health issues, it just meant that for the time being, I was more resilient. Soon enough though, I would discover that I wasn't as resilient as I thought I was.

By the time I was in my senior year, my mental health was at its worst. I had no means for coping with anything in a healthy way. I couldn't cope with anything emotionally and felt like I was totally on my own. I felt like there was no one to help me. I didn't want anyone to know how badly I was failing at being perfect, so asking for help or letting people in on the truth was out of the question. I didn't want to burden my parents with this, so I kept these thoughts to myself.

Right at the time when I was fully isolated with my dark thoughts and feelings, my brother got sick. He was having some digestive issues and had gone to see the doctor to discover why. The doctor diagnosed him with ulcerative colitis, a chronic, inflammatory bowel disease that causes inflammation in the digestive tract. He was prescribed a steroid to treat his illness. Unfortunately, his body was sensitive to steroids, and the extra release of insulin caused an onset of type 1 diabetes. He almost fell into a diabetic coma, but luckily, because of his age, he was able to survive through constant treatment and monitoring.

For almost an entire year, my family was in and out of the hospital with him. I was often left alone, sometimes the only one home to answer the door when people dropped off meal train meals that were meant to help us along. Accepting these meals left me feeling more shame for not eating them. When my parents did finally come home, they were rightfully concerned with managing my brother's new type 1 diabetes. This required him pricking his finger three times a day and checking his sugar numbers constantly. My parents feared that without constant monitoring, he could go into a coma. They did whatever it took to stay on top of his diet and insulin.

My needs went on the back burner. Because of my undernourishment and use of unhealthy dieting strategies, I was experiencing anxiety and low-level depression. I was getting myself ready to leave home and go off to college, but I was severely underprepared. I needed to learn how to become an adult, but I didn't know how to ask for more from my parents. I shoved my needs deep down and tried my best to live without any family support.

Restrictive dieting takes a huge toll on overall health. It leads to significant nutritional deficiencies, which can cause low energy, irritability, muscle weakness, hormone disruption, anxiety and depression. It can also worsen mental health because your brain isn't functioning optimally—and hunger can lead to poor impulse control, shame spirals and feelings of isolation. The super restrictive diet that I thought would solve all of my problems had actually created more. At the time though, I lacked the information and the support that I needed to get help.

4 I MISS FOOD

After high school graduation, I was set to go away to college in San Antonio. I was only moving two hours away from home, but it was the beginning of getting as far away from my old habits as possible. For starters, I couldn't starve myself for a minute longer. I wanted to eat. I missed food terribly. I wanted to eat tacos from some of the great taco places near my campus and I was ready to start drinking along with the new friends I was making, too. In college, eating and drinking were part of the lived experience; restriction was not. So I began to eat again, and food became my biggest comfort. I finally had my first taste of freedom. I wanted to eat, drink and be merry after so many years of feeling like food was my worst enemy. I'd been so restrictive for so long that I felt like I earned the right to have fun and let go of all the stress I'd been carrying. This was all I cared about.

If I'm being honest, in the very back of my mind, I was worried I would put weight back on. I began to negotiate with myself. When I wanted to go out drinking or eat a big serving of tacos, I would begin an inner negotiation. It would go something like this: *maybe I can skip breakfast and lunch, and only eat dinner and drink this evening*. If I knew a big night of drinking was ahead, I would think to myself *I will fast all day long*. This seemed like a reasonable plan to me. In fact, I believed that this plan of negotiating with myself was a very adult one. It was a big change from constant restriction and I felt like I was making progress. I figured that I was off to the races, finally getting a handle on my eating. I was learning how to be an adult. Or so I thought.

I was clueless when it actually came to maturity and being more adult-like. I hadn't learned how to balance a checkbook or pay bills. I didn't know how to self regulate, the process of monitoring your own thoughts, feelings and behaviors. I was completely unaware that feelings lead to thoughts which lead to actions. For example, when I was feeling low, I would sometimes reach for alcohol. It would help temporarily relieve my feelings of sadness or frustration, but in the end, it was inhibiting me from making any long term progress toward my overall goals. I just jumped from feelings to actions without any intentional thoughts of what might be best for my desired long-lasting goals or might provide me with the best outcome.

I went from a heavily monitored, highly structured life, under the pressure of my parents' watch at all times, to being out in the world with no supervision. Every decision was mine to make without having to consult a parent. Every choice was up to me. I had no experience with this and everything felt so new and exciting. I had restricted myself for so long and tried so hard to be perfect and yet still felt like I had failed miserably. This newfound freedom was my chance to not have to worry about everything so much, to let go of obsessing over every little thing I ate. I no longer had the structure and discipline that I had when I was at home, but instead of finding a more healthy balance, I just let it go completely by abandoning all structure and discipline.

The college environment couldn't have been further away from my neat, keep-it-together, perfect home environment. College was full of kids who wanted to party, stay up all night, sleep all day, go to class only when they felt like it—and it was a place where food was available at all times. Pizza places would deliver food in the middle of the night, the campus grill was always open and vending machine junk foods were the staples that college kids lived off of. From where I stood, it seemed that students were more focused on drinking and partying than they were studying, and that was just fine with me. I was finding that alcohol was the one thing that allowed me to let go. When I was drinking, the buzz I got helped stave off my buried obsession with my body.

My self esteem was still low. As I was seeking new friendships, I wound up seeking out people who weren't the best influence for my fragile self. They were emotionally unhealthy themselves, making negative choices when it came to overall well being. They too seemed to be abandoning structure and discipline. They would encourage me to cut class and go out drinking, or to go shopping and spend all of my money on new clothes.

Looking back, my weight going into college wasn't that bad. However, I felt that there was a standard that was set for me and that I needed to be perfect. When I felt that I failed to meet this standard (which was all the time) I began to think it wasn't my weight that was *bad*, it was just me that was *bad*. Because I felt that bad about myself, I projected that onto all my interactions. I had lots of negative self-talk, and made decisions that weren't good for my overall well-being (like skipping class to drink). Before long, the people around me started to treat me like I wasn't worthy. They began to reflect back to me what I already felt–unworthy. The chatter in my mind started up again and before I knew it, I was thinking things like,*Why bother studying when you are worthless? Why bother working hard when you're not good at anything? Why bother taking care of yourself when you're gaining weight so rapidly anyway?*

I was no longer playing sports, had zero adult supervision and was way too immature to understand exactly what it took to be an adult. I made one terrible choice after another. I stopped moving my body. After years of sports and over-exercising, it felt good to take a break and just allow myself to sit on the couch and watch TV. I was grasping desperately for comfort to cope with everything my family had been through with my brother, and to help me overcome the shame of who I had become throughout high school. I reached for anything externally that would give me that quick fix. This became food and drinks.

The dopamine hit that I would get after finishing a whole pizza was euphoric. Feelings and eating became intertwined, and soon I was using food to cope. When I was sad, I would go get a pint of ice cream. When I was bored, I would put on a movie and order a large pizza, finishing every last piece. When I wanted to let loose, I would drink, which would lead to even worse food choices and eating at all hours of the night. None of these habits happened every single day, but they happened enough that they were becoming a pattern and ultimately a way of life. Looking back, I find it ironic that just a year or so earlier, I despised gaining any amount of weight at all and restricted food at all costs—yet now that I was in college, I could find no other way to soothe myself than to eat and drink.

This was a time of difficult emotions for me. Being away from home, completely out of my element, and away from everyone I knew for the first time ever was something that I both loved and hated. I had freedom from all the schedules and activities I'd had in high school. I was learning how to navigate becoming a woman, but I couldn't navigate this well on my own. I still needed some structure so that I could learn how to make healthy choices for myself. I wasn't handling it well, and my anxiety and emotional expression really started to peak. Food became a way to hide hard feelings of discomfort or unresolved thoughts and emotions I felt incapable of expressing properly. I was hiding.

I joined a sorority. Having a group of girls around me and plenty of festive activities on my social calendar helped me avoid the fact that I was overeating and drinking. During holidays, the sorority would host all kinds of drinking and eating events to celebrate whatever was going on. There was a week in college around Halloween where I remember drinking for a whole week straight. We would start tailgating for the football game early in the day, which meant drinking in the morning. In the evening, there would be a Halloween party followed by an afterparty. When those parties ended, I visited some non-sorority friends who were hosting their own Halloween parties. I hopped from one party to the next, eating and drinking my way through each of them. The booze helped me keep my mind off of my body and it was so freeing. My friends and I started drinking on a Thursday night and just didn't stop. We soaked up our hang-overs with greasy food and started drinking again right away. This was normalized.

During that same week, I didn't pay my rent and I didn't go to any of my classes. I was in my apartment trying to recover from a night of drinking when I heard a knock at my door. I walked over, hoping it was a friend ready to give me the rundown on the events of the day, but when I opened the door, there stood my dad. "Why didn't you pay your rent?" he said, staring at me.

I didn't really know what to say. The truth was, I was finally having fun! I spent my rent money on booze and cute outfits to wear out to parties. When I wasn't obsessing about my body, it seems I let other things get out of my control too. I wasn't managing my money well at all.

I let him into my very small apartment feeling glad that it wasn't my mom who showed up. I was sure there was no way she would approve of how messy it was and how hungover I looked at this moment. He lovingly helped me clear things up by paying my overdue rent. I was appreciative and vowed that it was time to get my shit together—but not just yet. I still had some more partying to do first. I was in a rut, and I had no idea how to get myself out of it.

Looking back, I think I really believed that if I could just make it through that week, things would slow down. Once things slowed down a bit, I could try to go work out, eat better (or less) and take care of myself better for the next week. The problem was that the next week would end up being the very same. Drink, eat, party, repeat. These thoughts that I had like, *after this week, things will settle down* became an excuse that I would eventually live by for years. The reality was that things never did slow down. There was always going to be something going on. There would always be a party to go to, an invite that I couldn't turn down, dinner with friends, drinks to celebrate. I had rendered myself powerless to this new habitual cycle that would take root in my life for years to come.

One night, as I was getting ready to go out for a night of partying, I put on my usual pair of jeans and I couldn't zip them. With all the eating and drinking I'd been doing, I had started to gain some serious weight. I was slowly realizing that my relationship with food was unhealthy. The only thing I could think to do to comfort myself was to stay in, put on stretchy pants, order pizza and eat it all by myself. You would think that if your jeans didn't fit, the reverse would happen. But at this point in my life, food was my only way of coping. I had nothing else to soothe the devastation I was feeling. I remember thinking to myself, *this is the opposite direction of where you want to go Emily, just stop*. I would comfort the chatter in my mind with the same old phrase I was beginning to believe: *That's okay. I can have pizza tonight because tomorrow I'll change*. Only, I wouldn't wake up and suddenly change. The habits had formed and the patterns were set for me.

The true reason I wasn't obsessing about my body was because I was numb. I was doing something called *emotional eating*. Eating when emotionally hungry means that I was trying to fill the void, to numb the feelings of body hatred that I carried with me to college. I was using food to temporarily silence my uncomfortable emotions like shame, resentment, guilt and anxiety. When that didn't work, I washed it down with alcohol which helped me avoid all the feelings that I had been dealing with since adolescence. I wasn't at all free from my body dysmorphia. Instead, I was just kicking the can down the road, hoping to maintain the temporary relief that I so badly desired.

Overconsumption of food and alcohol can lead to depression and anxiety. Persistently drinking alcohol during emotional pain or stress may cause the opposite effect. "It comes down to the balance of neurotransmitters in your brain," says Dr. Joseph Volpicelli, executive director at the Institute of Addiction Medicine in Pennsylvania. "Alcohol increases your levels of GABA, a neurotransmitter that has a calming effect. Your brain responds to this increase by making more glutamate, increasing brain activity. As alcohol levels fall and GABA levels fall, the brain stays hyperactive from the extra glutamate activity." This could heighten symptoms such as anxiety. "To feel better, some people will drink alcohol the next day," he says. "Unfortunately, drinking alcohol to take away anxiety leads to a vicious cycle, in which drinking may lead you to want to drink more."[i]

Overeating comfort food instead of focusing on a healthy diet is also known to be a factor in developing depression, dementia and type 2 diabetes[ii]. Comfort foods can activate the reward centers in the brain. Foods high in sugar or foods that are highly processed mute the brain's ability to tell your body when it's satiated (like the "bliss point" I mentioned before). This leads to overeating foods that lack nutritional value even if you're not hungry. After binging, guilt often comes along, leaving a person with feelings of shame and resentment. If these feelings become too overwhelming, a person might look for something to numb these feelings, and then the cycle of overeating starts all over again.

I had unwittingly created a vicious cycle of using food and alcohol to cope, which then led me to want to eat and drink more. In addition, I'd gone from being active and playing sports to doing nothing. I wasn't moving my body very much and therefore wasn't getting any feel-good chemicals from exercise either.

I knew nothing about dopamine or other feel-good chemicals during this time in my life. I didn't know that you could get those feel-good chemicals through time spent in nature, walks, exercising and hanging out with friends in a way that doesn't center food and drink. Because food and alcohol was at the center of all of my social interactions, I didn't really know how to be in a social setting without it. There were so many rituals around food and beverages that became ingrained in my life. For example, having a drink on the airplane on the way to a vacation, letting loose on the weekends after a hard week of restriction or eating all the appetizers at Superbowl parties. It turned out I wasn't just going to have to reckon with my unhealthy food habits—I would also need to unlearn the habit of using food to cope and socialize.

I ate and drank my way through college, prolonging any progress with my unhealthy relationship with food. But as I got a little older, graduated and got my first job, things started to change. I was growing more responsible. Slowly and over time, I learned to do adult things like pay bills, and I started to gain some progress on my eating and drinking (if only because I wanted to look better in my jeans).

I joined a gym and started to move my body again. It felt good to do CrossFit and yoga, and I liked being a part of a community of people who prioritized fitness in the way that I had as a child. Having a job and joining a gym helped put the much-needed structure back into my life. There were places that I needed to be at certain times, which meant I would need to be somewhat responsible outside of those times in order to make that work. I liked having structure again. Things began feeling less chaotic. I began to restrict my food again, but not as severely as before (no diet pills or laxatives this time around), and I cut back on drinking alcohol throughout the weekdays since I had work in the morning and workout classes at night. I would start on the new fad diet of the season and was able to drop twenty pounds here and there only to gain it all back again once I stopped the diet. It wasn't a great cycle, but it was healthier than the restriction in high school and the all-out bingeing in college. I felt like I was doing better overall, both emotionally and physically.

I started to become really close with my new CrossFit friends. During the week as a collective group, we would be as "good" as we could. Then when the weekend rolled around, the plan was always to have drinks and dinner somewhere after our workout Friday, then to watch college football at a bar on Saturday. We'd start at noon and watch until 8 o'clock at night, which included eating twice wherever we were. We drank most of that time too. On Sundays, some of us might start to detox, but others would just keep going. Maybe we would go to a park or be open to whatever amazing Sunday adventure was happening in downtown Houston.

Mondays were for detoxing. This meant no drinking, no overeating or even eating out, doing hard workouts and then wash, rinse and repeat. Most weekdays, I would restrict food, exercise a lot and "white-knuckle" through the week until the weekend rolled around. On the weekend, I could finally let go, eat whatever I felt like eating, drink as much as I wanted and start it all over again on Monday.

While it's normal for weekend eating/drinking to look a little different than eating/drinking during the week because of change in our routines, this type of restriction/binge was not healthy. During the week, almost every minute of my day was scheduled. I worked a lot of hours starting early in the morning and didn't get home until later in the evening. I would then hit the gym, cook dinner, take a shower and go to bed. I had to get up early and do it all over again the next day. Weekends were different. Most of the things that I had to do were "fun" things, which usually meant that there would be an array of eating and drinking activities. Things like a girls night out with dinner or tailgating for the football game followed by drinks to celebrate the win. I had already worked out so hard during the week that I would give myself days off of working out on the weekends, too. I could sleep in, which meant being less worried about a hangover, and my plan was always to reel it all back in by Sunday night.

Today, there is more information about why these types of binge/restrict diets don't work. In fact, many experts say that restriction may be the single biggest factor on whether or not a person will binge. Consequences of this type of lifestyle usually result in preoccupation with your body and food (which I had already experienced for most of my life), mental health issues, lack of progress toward maintaining a healthy weight and hormone disruption.

Restricting your diet actually causes a lot of stress on your body. Your body loves homoeostasis, which is balance. You can best achieve this balance through consistency. When you have a very low calorie intake during the week and then huge binges on the weekends, it causes your body to get dysregulated. You then have large blood sugar upswings because you're eating more fat and more carbohydrates, which are both like quick burning fuel. This will cause your blood sugar to become low quickly, and then cause huge blood sugar downswings which are hard for your body to process. This creates stress and inflammation within your body.

The greatest thing that you can do for yourself is eat in a consistent manner so blood sugar can stay regulated. Your body can work to get the nutrients that you are eating to the proper organs and functions in a really sustainable way. When you restrict and binge like I was, you just do not have enough food or fuel during the week, and then your body has to break down a large amount of food on the weekends.

When you have these moments of dysregulation and your body gets super-stressed, the restriction/binge lifestyle can cause a lot of different metabolic functions to go wrong. You can put stress on your heart. You can put stress on your hormones, which affects your mood. Once your hormones are imbalanced and dysregulated, it can cause your gut to have major issues so that you won't absorb nutrients properly. This eating style can cause a myriad of issues over time like autoimmune disease and poor cardiovascular health.

I didn't know or care about my overall well-being at the time. I just wanted to be thin, and as I was in my twenties, it was a more forgiving time. Usually, during our twenties, our bodies have a higher metabolism, we have more muscle mass and we have fewer responsibilities. If a slip-up occurred, I could just get right back to restricting food or spend extra time in the gym. I didn't have kids depending on me and my hormone levels were more naturally balanced despite my destructive habits. Beneath the surface, there was a lot more going on. This lifestyle was priming me for what was to come–the onset of PPD.

My life was feeling more stable and my mental health was under control even though I was living a binge/restrict/binge lifestyle. I was in a serious relationship with my partner and pretty soon after that, we got married. This changed my life in a lot of ways. Marriage gave me a type of role that I'd never had before. I was now responsible for someone else's feelings and not just my own. We shared agendas, finances, decisions about what we ate, where we would travel and more. This type of relationship helped me mature. I was now thinking about someone else's needs.

My spouse was very health-conscious. He was a college athlete. His approach to wellness was about finding the balance between proper nutrition and exercise. He had a working knowledge of how getting enough protein, eating fruits and vegetables and reducing carbohydrates could improve overall health. When we met, he was in incredible shape, and eating healthy was important to him. It was the first time that I realized that nutrition could really play a role in your health. His eating style had nothing to do with the newest fad diet, severe restriction or hours of exercise a day.

Due to his emphasis on nutrition, we began cooking together

and started to eat most meals at home during the week. There was less fast food than I was used to when I was single, and much less drinking, too. We really only drank on the weekends, and it was much more responsible than it had been in college. I hadn't had this element of structure in a long time, and it felt good to me. It helped me find clarity in other things, too.

At the time, I was working in mortgage sales. That wasn't what I set out to do exactly—it was just the first job that I landed out of college. It started feeling less desirable as the days went on. I felt like I was meant to do more with my life.

I had studied early childhood education in college, and when I found out that I could take exams to get my teaching degree, I knew this is what I wanted to do. Both of my parents were teachers, and so were so many of the people that I loved. Teaching felt like a job that I could be proud of, a way to make a bigger impact on the world. I really loved working with kids and it felt natural to me after all those years of watching my parents do it. I knew that getting into public education could make a true impact on lives, and I was ready to go for it. I studied for the exams for twelve weeks, passed both and got my teaching degree. I felt really proud of myself for this accomplishment, and I knew that this was going to be the right career path for me.

Things were really falling into place, and I felt more mature than I ever had. I hadn't made a lot of progress toward my nutrition, and my mental health was still unstable, but I was learning things about myself that would help me later on in life. I liked structure and routine, and needed both of those things in my life to be successful. Structure and routine helped me feel stable, and it put a stop to both the starvation and the binge eating. I still had a lot to learn in terms of how to properly nourish my mind, body and soul but I was developing the structure that I needed to feel successful in some areas of my life.

5 AS MY BELLY GREW, SO DID MY PROBLEMS

THROUGHOUT MY LATE TWENTIES, I WAS GAINING LIFE EXPERIENCE and felt like I was becoming more mature. I had more stability, a healthy marriage, enough money to pay the bills, a job that I loved and the overall feeling that I had finally arrived at adulthood. I was growing up and the older I got, the more mature I felt. Most of my friends had started to have babies, and I knew that having a family was something that I wanted. But I had this deep feeling inside of me that I needed more time to mature before having kids. There was still so much that I needed to learn about adulting before I could bring a child into this world. I took the time I needed to learn how to live a more stable life. I waited until I was thirty-three to get pregnant with our first child.

While I had grown in so many ways in terms of learning to be responsible, I was still struggling with my nutrition. By the time I became pregnant with my first baby, my relationship with food was toxic. My body was primed for a hormone meltdown and the onset of depression. I had spent my whole life either starving or binging. Little did I know the toll the years of binging and restricting had taken on my body's entire system, and that this was going to be escalated by pregnancy hormones.

Regardless, I had high hopes for my pregnancy. For starters, I was able to get my body in great shape right before I got pregnant. I wanted to go into pregnancy looking lean and feeling good about my weight. I had already decided that I was going to have a goal of losing all of the baby weight and getting right back into my thin body as soon as the baby was born! I had a plan to continue to work out during my pregnancy and to restrict food (as long as the baby was healthy) so that I didn't gain too much weight.

Unfortunately, my plans were going to have to wait. As soon as I got pregnant, I developed a sickness that would last throughout my entire pregnancy. I was completely blindsided by nausea. I began throwing up three times a day, and this lasted for the entirety of my pregnancy. There were times when I knew I was going to be sick and could make it to the bathroom; other times, it came out of nowhere. I started carrying throw-up bags in my car and would often use them when driving to work in the morning.

I had never experienced any kind of sickness like this before. If you've never been debilitated by sickness, it's impossible to understand how it can slow down your life and aggravate anything you typically love to do. Just managing your sickness takes over your entire life. You have no room, time or space for anything else. I remember thinking to myself that I never knew that someone could feel this bad and still try to manage their day-to-day life. I will always carry an affinity for anyone living in chronic pain or with any type of health concern that gets in the way of their daily functioning.

During this time, I was a first grade teacher, and just getting to work was a job within itself. I would drag myself into my classroom feeling completely nauseous and yet responsible for so many small children who were depending on me. I would do my best to get through each lesson, sometimes having to run to the restroom and get sick. I would return and do the best that I could, looking forward to the time of day when the students left my classroom to go to music or art. As soon as the students would leave, I would lay down on the floor of my classroom and try not to die. I had very little time before they would return, and there was nothing I could do to feel better other than to not move a muscle.

One day as I lay on the floor taking deep breaths, my eyes red and watery from both throwing up and crying, I thought to myself: *well, this is definitely not what I expected to feel like when I thought about pregnancy*. That old familiar feeling of *why can't you just be normal like everyone else?* started creeping back in. Here I was, thinking that pregnancy would be the joyful experience I had heard other women talking about all my life. I began to believe deeply that something must be wrong with me. I was not aware that bringing life into this world would also be painful and exhausting. Why had no one ever mentioned this before? I was also not aware (or lacked the emotional intelligence that I have now) to understand that two truths can exist at once. I could be excited and eager to bring a child into this world and I could also resent the fact that I was feeling sick all of the time.

This was going to be a journey for me. I was going to have to learn the lesson that life is about paradoxes. I could experience joy, but it could also go hand in hand with pain and discomfort. That did not mean that there was something wrong with me. In fact, what I was feeling was incredibly normal. All parts of me needed to be given importance and space to feel. At the time, I wasn't aware of any of this. I just assumed that any negative feelings I had during my pregnancy meant that I was already failing at being a mother.

During this time, I didn't see things in a clear way—it felt as if I just couldn't thrive. In fact, thriving was out of the question. I was barely surviving. All I could think about was the end of my pregnancy and getting this baby out of me so that I could function again. At every doctor's appointment, I would ask how early was too early for the baby to come. I would daydream about no longer being pregnant and therefore, no longer sick.

I did this sort of daydreaming frequently. I always assumed

that if I could just get "there"—to the other side of whatever very hard thing I was experiencing right then—everything would be better, and I would be free of emotional distress. Sadly, this was an unhealthy pattern for me. This type of thinking ends up causing us more distress because there is no arrival point. Instead, there is only opportunity to refine your perspective in the present moment you are in. You will never get to where you want to go until you embrace what you need to experience and understand in the here and now.

I stopped moving altogether and started eating any and every food that would bring me comfort. Old habits die hard. I hadn't healed anything about my eating habits from my earlier years. I had learned to eat healthier in order to look good, but I still lacked coping skills or any real strategies for self regulation. I still didn't have any larger community or support around a healthy lifestyle, and I hadn't done any emotional work. As soon as I started feeling bad, I fell back on the only thing I knew, that food equals comfort. This meant that I was back to eating processed foods—and just like before my pregnancy, I couldn't have cared less about my calorie intake.

I remember feeling really isolated during this time. I was triggered by other moms who seemed to love being pregnant. A few of my friends already had babies, and I remembered going to their baby showers or seeing them socially while they were pregnant. They were glowing and looked happy. Their bodies didn't seem to be working against them. I didn't hear them complaining of morning sickness or feelings of nausea. This made me feel frustrated, another way in which I felt like I must be doing something wrong. *What is wrong with me that I can't have a normal pregnancy?* Instead, I felt like I had the chronic flu and that I was sinking.

One day, I was standing in the kitchen eating an entire German chocolate cake—the weight gain by that point was incredible, and I had completely lost all control.

"You know that doesn't come out with the baby, right?" My

husband joked. This was not a joke I wanted to hear at that moment. But it was probably the exact thing I needed to hear. It wasn't about the cake, it was about me desperately trying to find a way to numb myself. What I wished he'd said was *you cannot numb yourself anymore, Emily, and hide from the things that are happening in this present moment. This will only make you more sick.* I wish I knew at the time that releasing emotions and having boundaries with yourself is actually incredibly healthy.

At our doctor's appointments, I remember telling my husband that I would kill him if he told anyone the number on the scale. But one appointment in particular was monumental for me, and I will never forget it. The number was larger than I had ever seen before. Seeing it immediately took me back to the moment in junior high when my weight was written down on the clipboard and I was heavier than most of the kids in my class. My weight was now more than my husband's. I was humiliated. The embarrassment from this was all too consuming.

I assumed I'd get the weight off when the baby came. I thought I would be able to start working on my body again, exercise again and eat healthy right away. I had no idea what was coming and that this goal would be nearly impossible to achieve.

In between getting sick and trying to survive, I did spend some time learning things that I thought were important. I was reading all the recommended books like *What To Expect When You're Expecting,* and googling which crib and baby monitor would keep my baby the safest. Unfortunately, I don't remember hearing a single word about mental and physical health during maternity. If I'd looked harder, there may have been books or articles, but I didn't even know I should be looking for this kind of information. It just wasn't on my radar. At the time, caring for your maternal mental health just wasn't a social norm. My doctor wasn't talking to me about the proper nutrition to keep me and the baby healthy. No one was encouraging me to keep moving, and this would have been impossible anyway, given my sickness. There were no books about PPD, or how to manage or avoid feelings of isolation. This is unfortunate, because there is plenty of research now regarding fluctuating hormones and how these can have an impact on maternal mental health.

By this point in my pregnancy, I'd gained 65 pounds. When I was triggered by feeling mentally unbalanced, I would turn to food. This wasn't necessarily because I was hungry, but because numbing had become a way of life. It was a pattern that I would return to consistently whenever feelings of discomfort would arise. I didn't know at the time that it was okay for me to feel "undesirable" emotions of sadness, anxiety, frustration and anger. I thought experiencing these negative feelings was a bad thing—so as soon as they came on, I tried to bury them. I never allowed them to move through me. I never allowed myself to learn how to feel. I only numbed.

When my baby girl was born, I did get relief from feeling physically sick, but it was soon replaced by the overwhelming chronic fatigue of being a new mother. This was such a key point for me to learn, that there is a pattern we can see emerging in all of our lives. There will always be something else that exhausts you, depletes you, surprises you or something that makes life difficult. We cannot manage a life where we believe things like *as soon as I get to point A, everything will be okay*. It is much more complicated than that. Instead, what we need to learn is how to embrace where we are, and get curious as to how we can show up best now. Whatever season we may find ourselves in, that is the invitation, and that is the gift.

I hadn't learned any of this yet. I was still trying to get rid of negativity at all costs. *Once I get through this hard thing,* I thought, *my life will be waiting for me.*

Caring for a newborn is one of the most difficult things I have ever done in my life. It wasn't what I expected, and I was shocked at the amount of pressure on me to keep my baby alive. I was nursing exclusively, which led to significant sleep deprivation. The burden of being the only parent who could feed our baby was huge. My spouse could help with diaper changes and things like house cleaning, but the baby spent most of her time wanting to nurse, which meant that I was her primary caretaker. The immense pressure felt unbearable at times, given my lack of sleep.

That level of sleep deprivation was a shock to my system. Even in the hospital, after just giving birth, I asked the nurse to take the baby so I could just rest for a few moments. I'd only been a mom for a few hours but I was already exhausted. When the nurse came in to check on us, I mustered up the courage I needed to ask for help. "Is there any way that you can take her to the nursery so that I could rest for just a little while?" I asked sheepishly.

"Sure!" she said, as she took my baby carefully and walked her out of the room. In that moment of peace, I began to let my eyes rest. It was just a minute or so before I heard the door opening again.

"She won't stop crying," the nurse told me as she approached, handing my baby right back to me.

I felt completely overwhelmed. Here I was, a new mom, and I wanted to follow the rules. The hospital made it very clear that it was dangerous to allow your baby to sleep on your chest. I couldn't get my baby to stop crying. And now, neither could the professionals? My only choice was to not sleep. I wondered how in the world I was going to figure this out. I can remember a feeling of panic. I asked myself *Does anyone know how to do this?*

I struggled to cope with the stress of not sleeping and began to feel like a failure. That morning, my friend came to visit us and see the baby. I was totally naked with my robe unbuttoned, walking around the hospital room. She came in and asked, "How was last night?"

I broke down in tears and she seemed surprised. I looked noticed that she looked fresh , showered and so full of life. It made me feel even worse about myself. Just a day or two ago, I would have been showered and fresh, which now seemed like an impossible task. I wasn't sure what else to say. I apologized over and over for my breakdown, and tried as best I could to seem optimistic for the rest of the visit. Again, my old thinking pattern took hold. *Why couldn't I get it together like other moms?*

The emotional pain I was experiencing wasn't registering at first. I was so happy to not be throwing up and was too overwhelmed with exhaustion to notice that I was starting to feel off. In quiet moments, though, I noticed a feeling within me that was unsettling. I knew I wasn't feeling as excited as my other mom friends about having a newborn. I avoided this feeling by telling myself that I was just too tired. It seemed to me that other moms were coping fine on no sleep, so I didn't mention how tired I felt out of fear of being judged. Being a mom was just another area for me to compare myself to others. Whether or not they were thriving better than I was or happy with the transition to motherhood was not actually something I could have known because I didn't have the energy or the mental space to ask.

When we're suffering, it can seem as though everyone else is not. It was only after I healed that I became brave enough to have conversations with many moms. I would learn that we were all struggling in some way, shape or form. I was never alone. It became apparent to me how much we need each other—and how important it is to express ourselves and let more love and gratitude in. But I could only begin to feel this way once I stopped numbing myself and began to process my difficult emotions.

I now know that a difficult pregnancy followed by a difficult baby are both indicators of increased risk for PPD. Nobody I knew was talking about PPD, though. I didn't have a support group or a community openly talking about these truths. I thought that what I was experiencing was a bout of the "baby blues." This was something that people often referred to when talking about new moms who felt tired and weary. The feelings I was having totally sucked, but I thought they were part of motherhood.

I was struggling to function. There was a time when my daughter had a horrible diaper rash. She was taking antibiotics which caused her to have acidic diarrhea that lasted for days and left her little bottom raw and bleeding. The only place she would relax was in a hot bath. I could not figure out how to help her and it felt like we were in crisis. My lack of sleep, coupled with my desperation to end my daughter's pain, left me feeling illogical. I felt the exclusive burden, that I alone must do something about this. So I lay there with the baby on my chest, holding her little butt cheeks open so that she could properly air out. I thought this was the only solution to this problem. When my friend stopped by and saw this, she was stunned.

"Emily, you don't have to hold her like that," she said.

"What else can I do?" I asked in desperation.

She kindly offered me some proper diaper cream that was thicker and more healing than regular creams, similar to something they used in the hospital. The support I received from my friend that day was invaluable. I needed someone to understand how urgent this was for me and offer me guidance and help. The weight of motherhood was becoming heavy, but on that day I, didn't have to do it alone.

This is something else I would learn over time while working through all of my mental health struggles. When you are in this type of mental space, it feels like there are no options for you besides the one you see. Today, whenever I feel stuck, it is a great indicator to me that I need a break, either to nurture myself or to seek support from someone to help me feel safe and find stable ground. Taking a break or getting help will help you detach. When you step back from a situation, you see there are always options. You are not trapped in the emotions you are feeling—you just may need some tools to move through them. This is a practice I maintain even today.

I was six months postpartum when I went to see my OBGYN for a check-up. I had noticed some things that were concerning me. My hair had started to fall out, my energy was extremely low (even though my daughter had finally started sleeping through the night), and when I stepped on the scale, the number never moved, no matter what I did the day before. I felt swollen all over. I asked the doctor to check my thyroid.

"That's not something you really need at this point," she replied. "Your regular blood work should be enough."

"I understand." I said, "But I just don't feel right at all. Is there any way that we can just please check it?" I pleaded.

(Note here for all readers: Trust your gut no matter what the experts say. You are and always will be your biggest advocate.)

She agreed to check my thyroid. The next day I got a voicemail that she needed to talk to me ASAP. I knew something was up because doctors don't usually leave that kind of message. I called back right away. She explained to me that my TSH (thyroid-stimulating hormone) was very high, which was an indicator that I had an underactive thyroid. I was so glad that I advocated for myself and got the testing that I needed. I discovered that I had Hashimoto's disease.

Hashimoto's disease, or Hashimoto's thyroiditis, is a condition that leads to hypothyroidism. This occurs when the butterfly-shaped thyroid gland in the front of the neck is unable to produce enough thyroid hormones, causing the bodily functions to slow down. These hormones regulate metabolism, muscle strength, body temperature and many other vital processes. Hashimoto's disease is the most common cause of hypothyroidism. Low thyroid function can cause weight gain, lower cardiac fitness and irregular heart rhythms among a host of other issues.

I didn't know this at the time, but having thyroid issues is common after pregnancy. So much about pregnancy relates to your autoimmune system. Your hormones all need to be working properly during pregnancy and while giving birth. When they're not, hormonal imbalances can start to have an impact on your entire system, especially your thyroid. I started treatment right away, but I felt like I was breaking.

One night, I was lying in bed and started sweating profusely. I felt hot to the touch, so I got up and took my temperature. It was 104 degrees. I never remembered having a temperature this high. I didn't have any other symptoms and it came on so fast. As I lay in bed sweating, a thought crossed my mind: *Am I pregnant?*

My spouse and I knew we wanted to have a large family. We both wanted at least two kids, if not more. It took a while for me to get pregnant with our first child. One night when our daughter was a little over a year old, we were sitting around doing the math. We decided that if we wanted to have our kids two years apart and it would take at least six months to conceive, we should start trying soon. We didn't have a way to track ovulation because I was still nursing and hadn't yet gotten my period back. We started trying anyway.

At the time, I felt a lot of pressure and anxiety about pregnancy. It had been so hard the first time around that I just wanted to "get it over with." I hadn't yet completely healed, but I figured I might as well do it now while I was still in the thick of it. It was also very important to me that my baby had a sibling. I wanted her to have someone else in the world that she could count on. I wanted her to know that she wasn't alone with just us, her parents. That mindset was what pushed all other logic (and thoughts like *I'm feeling pretty awful, why not wait a little longer?*) to the back burner.

We began to try again and unlike my first pregnancy, I got pregnant immediately. The reality of the situation was mind-numbing. In nine months, I would have two babies under the age of two. *How could I possibly do this?* I thought. I would calm myself down by thinking things like, *how bad could it be? My brother and I were 17 months apart; this is what my kids will be. This is doable.*

I shared the news with my spouse and he was happy. We were going to have that big family that we both wanted! He felt more relaxed and at ease than I did. Other than changing diapers, these babies didn't interrupt his life at all, or at least not in the ways they seemed to disrupt life for me. I am sure he struggled in different ways, but all I could see were the physical demands on me to bring life into the world. He didn't have to carry them in his womb or stay awake all night feeding them from his body. I was going to be the one who experienced the brunt of this giant responsibility. I was having a great pity party.

I also started feeling a lot of guilt about robbing my first baby of precious time that she needed from me. Getting pregnant so soon meant that I would have to stop nursing sooner than I had planned. This made me feel like I was already failing at meeting the expectations that I had set for myself. My feelings about having a second baby so soon were not that positive. I was worried that I wouldn't be able to meet the expectations required of me. I wanted to be the best mom that I could be, and having two babies so close together was going to be more of a challenge than I had ever faced. But this was happening; I was pregnant while caring for a baby.

Luckily, I wasn't as nauseous the second time around and I didn't throw up as often. The physical sickness, though, was quickly replaced by the overwhelming dread of what would soon become my reality. Taking care of a baby while pregnant was not easy. No one around me really seemed to be recognizing this monumental task. Everyone seemed to be going about their normal lives. For me, though, it was hard to enjoy life, let alone thrive when I was the sole responsible human keeping two babies alive. The pressure was crushing.

I remember suddenly feeling really angry at my mom. She had my brother and I seventeen months apart. I don't recall her ever saying a single word about how hard pregnancy was when you had a baby at home. She made the whole thing look easy! Her ease was what led me to believe that I could do this, too. At the time, it didn't occur to me that I was almost 10 years older than my mom was when she was dealing with two babies.

My solution to the strong feelings I was having was to place the blame on others instead of owning it myself. Unfortunately, this led to more suffering. My imagination would lead me to so much negativity. I let anger fuel me. It wasn't long before things started to get very dark. I would have long crying spells and felt extremely irritable. I was very overwhelmed all of the time, but didn't want anyone to come over to help me. I was completely isolated and nothing made me feel excited or happy. It's ironic that at the time I needed the most help, I isolated myself further. I began to question whether or not I should have had kids at all. I started wondering what the point of anything was. I wouldn't answer my phone if people called. Life in general, down to the smallest of tasks, felt hard. I had surrounded myself with a fortress whose walls were so thick that I was unable to allow the love I needed in.

Being pregnant while caring for a baby was a new kind of effort and exhaustion for me when I already felt so low. I couldn't just lie down when I felt tired or go on a walk when I needed one. I had to be a mom, which frequently meant not taking care of myself. I would give everything I had to keep the baby alive, and when she finally went to sleep at night, I would just fall apart.

One night, I handed our crying daughter to my husband. "Here, you take her," I said. "I'm going to Mexico," We both laughed, but deep down, I wasn't joking. I knew that I wanted to walk out. I wanted to leave it all behind. I couldn't take the pain of the depression and feelings of failure any longer.

I finally told my husband how I felt. I explained to him that I hadn't had a single positive thought in months and that I didn't feel connected—warm and fuzzy—with the baby. I felt like a zombie and my thoughts were going dark. Thoughts like: *What if I leave and don't come back? I'm a failure as a mother. I'm never going to be able to be a good mother. I'm not cut out for this.* I couldn't see a brighter side or step back from these feelings of despair.

I was eight months pregnant.

I was not suicidal, but I didn't want to do *it* anymore, and that scared me. I didn't want to do any of it: be a mom, take care of my baby, take care of my body or anything at all that required any energy from me. I had nothing left. I wanted my life, but was this the beginning of having suicidal-like thoughts. I didn't want to be a mom anymore. I didn't think I could take care of my kids. This rocked my boat. All I ever heard leading up to motherhood is that it is a gift and you're supposed to love every moment of it. Or at least that was all I thought I was hearing. I must have blocked out that anything bad could possibly come from motherhood. Maybe I was disillusioned into believing that if I could just have *this* or be *this* or experience *this*, my life would begin and I would be happy.

Regardless, this wasn't what I thought it would be. I was struggling with the fact that I was put on this earth to procreate and have a happy life, and I just wasn't. I felt like I was broken. I wanted to quit. I wanted to give up and just hand my baby back to the hospital because, at that moment, I figured somebody else could probably do it better. Those thoughts really scared me.

Now that I had let my husband know how bad I felt, we both agreed that getting help was the next step. I didn't know where to look for help, but I reached out to my friend who worked at a very well-respected women's health department in a hospital. She put me in touch with a psychiatrist who specialized in post-partum health. I drove to the office feeling a small glimmer of hope. I was desperate and I wanted answers.

I sat in her office, which looked like any normal therapist's office. I had a box of tissues in my lap. I sat on the couch across from her and let it all out. I told her I was desperate, isolated and that I didn't like being a mother. I told her that I had no positive thoughts and that I had scary thoughts of leaving my baby behind. I completely spilled it all. I said things that I didn't even have words for.

"I don't know how to not be sad anymore," I said as I cried and wiped my face with a tissue.

She was quiet and let me go on.

"I wish I could give my baby back to the hospital. I know other moms don't feel like this. Or at least not good moms. There's something wrong with me," I wailed.

She sat there taking notes and nodding her head. I noticed that she didn't seem alarmed. Was she not hearing me? I had just told her that I don't want my children–as I sat there eight months pregnant with a baby at home–and she barely batted an eye. I didn't know if this was because she didn't care, or because she had seen so much of this that it didn't phase her. Looking back, I realize that maybe she was holding space for me. But all I knew was this was shocking to me. I expected her to say, "Oh my! This won't do! We deem you unfit to continue on," or something like that. Regardless, I felt more isolated. While my whole world was crumbling down, other people were going on like normal.

"You have prenatal depression, which is depression that resulted from your first pregnancy and went untreated," she explained. "This will not go away on its own. In fact, at about six weeks after giving birth, you will have another hormone shift that will result in more severe PPD symptoms if you let this go untreated."

I was stunned. I didn't get what I needed. I thought that this was going to be something that I could control. I thought that a few months postpartum, I would start getting regular sleep and begin to feel normal again. Now this doctor was suggesting that that wouldn't happen. She went on to explain that I'd probably feel better once I returned to work. I think she meant that once I had time away from the babies, I would feel like my old self again. But I didn't see that as a viable long-term solution.

At this point, women's health was severely understudied, and no one really knew much about PPD. Even though I was seeing the top doctor in the state of Texas, her recommendations were antiquated. Today, things are more clear, and there's more of a national conversation surrounding PPD. There are many ways to reduce the symptoms of PPD without medication. Exercise, carving time out away from the babies, getting adequate sleep and eating a diet (like a Mediterranean diet) that consists of Omega-3 fatty acids/fish oil can greatly reduce the severity of PPD. My doctor didn't go over any of those options with me. I was going to need to decide for myself the things that I needed to do.

Since it had been so long since I had done any kind of self care, I wanted to start there. I wanted to see how far I could get on my own before trying medical interventions. I knew medication might be necessary, and for many people, it is a wonderful plan. I prepared myself to do whatever it took to get well, but I wanted to first see what I could do naturally. I knew in the back of my mind that if this got further away from me than I could handle, I would do whatever it took to get better and create a plan that worked for me.

I left the doctor's office with a filled prescription (just in case I needed it) and a new understanding of what it was going to take to get well, feeling both discouraged and enlightened. I knew that I must address my mental illness.

After finally revealing my true feelings and struggles, I felt like a slight weight was lifted. I had told a doctor my most horrible truth and nothing *bad* really happened at all. No one came to take the baby away. My husband was still supportive and didn't regret that I was the mother of our children. My baby was in perfect health, and although my thoughts were dark, my interactions with her were pure and kind. I wasn't completely failing. As I walked to my car, I was letting go of something—the heavy burden that I would somehow ruin it all. The truth had somehow set me free. When I finally reached out and asked for help, it eased the psychological stress that I was suffering with in isolation. I was no longer alone in this.

I called my friend.

"Hey," I said when she answered. "I just left the doctor. I've got PPD and it's not looking good."

"Oh no," she said worriedly. "What are you going to do about it?" she asked.

"I'm gonna change my whole fucking life," I told her.

"What do you mean?" she asked.

"I don't know exactly," I said. "But everything is going to change."

I had no choice but to begin to heal. Nobody was coming to save me. This moment was the beginning of a profound journey I was about to embark on, one in which I would begin to transform my inner person and find the freedom I had always been looking for. I can look back now and have such gratitude for what my kids have given me; love, compassion and a soul that would finally figure out how to let go and come alive.

It really made me curious that I was only offered medication that day, rather than a plan on how to change my life outside of that. I couldn't justify taking the medication—especially since I was eight months pregnant and I wasn't sure how this would impact the baby—when I hadn't so much as gone on a walk to try to feel better.

I knew after speaking to the psychiatrist that it was either medication or as much support as I could possibly render to help me get through this. I knew that PPD was not something that I was going to be able to beat alone. As soon as I got home, I started talking with my husband about what I needed. After a lifetime of depending on no one but myself, it took a lot of bravery for me to finally ask for help. Looking back, I feel really proud of myself for being able to recognize the importance of this. I give myself a lot of credit for mustering up the courage to do what needed to be done. This has allowed me to gain the skills necessary to do this in every phase and season of my life.

PART TWO

"You will not always be motivated so you must learn to be disciplined."

– Author unknown

6 IF NOTHING CHANGES, NOTHING CHANGES

After leaving the doctor's appointment, something inside me shifted. I knew that I was going to change, even though everything in my environment was the same. The advice from the doctor, that I was not going to get better on my own, was the most loving thing she could have possibly told me. It showed me that I needed to seek out help.

Let me tell you, help is what changed my life and continues to do so. I felt I had no choice; my babies needed me. It was almost like a spiritual revelation. I had found the inner strength it was going to take to walk a road I had never walked before, to be someone I had never been before. It was non-negotiable for me. Leaving that appointment, I suddenly had the energy and strength to show up in a way I had never experienced before.

In an essay written in the *Pharmacy Times,* author Anyssa Garza reviewed a study that showed there is evidence that both persistent and severe postpartum depression increases the risk of adverse outcomes in children. Research has found an association between postpartum depression and delayed cognitive and language development, disorganized or insecure attachment, higher rates of behavioral problems and lower grades. In addition, there is a documented link between postpartum depression and higher rates of depression in children during the latter teen years (16 to 18 years old).[i]

In addition to postpartum depression being an indicator of childhood mental health and learning problems, there are also some scary statistics on the maternal mortality rate as a result of PPD. Postpartum depression is the leading cause of maternal mortality—23% of pregnancy-related deaths, including suicide, are related to a mental health crisis.[ii] Research is finding that some of the worst outcomes for women occur up to a year after giving birth. Frustratingly, a CDC study shows that health care providers are missing opportunities to ask pregnant and postpartum people about feelings of depression. According to the study, about 1 in 5 pregnant people were not asked about symptoms of depression during a prenatal visit. About 1 in 8 people were not asked during a postpartum visit.[iii]

This was true in my case. But I was about to embark on something empowering and inspiring. I was about to show up and heal my story so that my kids and I all had a chance to thrive in this world. Showing up for yourself during a hard season is something that heals everyone around you. I had to discover treatment for myself after suffering for months.

I now understood that my condition was serious and would not go away on its own. I had finally reached a point of desperation, a point where continuing on my current path was harder than changing my behavior. This can be such a great thing. When you no longer have what it takes to stay stuck anymore, you can find yourself. This is the place of true change. It has to come from the depths of your own soul, where the pain of where you are is far greater than the pain of what you will endure on the road to change.

Desperation breeds survival. I had to connect to my most compelling reason for why this change mattered to me. Why? Because if I didn't change, my kids were going to have an exhausted, resentful mom who lacked the energy to properly care for them. I was already living my life with zero energy, watching the hours on the clock tick by until it was bedtime, when I could finally lay down and have time to myself. I did not want to be the kind of mom that doesn't have energy to engage with her kids. They deserved better than that. I owed it to them to show up.

I'm not sure I would have changed if it was just for me, but having them gave me the motivation to wake up to the life that I wanted. And later, through the process of showing up for my babies, I would discover something even more powerful. I was worth showing up for. I stumbled into beauty along the way and recognized it was *me* who was worth saving.

But how do you change when you're so far away from the person that you want to become or get back to? I was lost. After so many years of unhealthy eating habits and poor self-esteem, I didn't have a strong foundation that I could look back upon to guide me. I was starting from scratch, and I was going to need a lot of help.

How do you change your whole life and become a fit-minded person from the inside out? These were questions that I had to ask myself, and I was curious to find out. Curiosity is the foundation of learning, and learning produces change. When you know better, you do better. Sometimes we just need better skills and tools in order to make life-changing decisions.

I tell my clients who are just starting out that finding the reason why you want to change is your first task. If you do not have a compelling reason, you might not be able to do what it takes to change—especially if you have never done anything like this before or don't trust yourself to be able to do it. Your why is what keeps you going when you feel like giving up. My why was my kids.

In working with hundreds of women, I've learned that we all reach points in our lives (sometimes multiple times) where seasons shift and change is necessary. In order to live a meaningful life, you have to come back to yourself in new ways and find your reasons why as these shifts happen. As seasons and cycles change, so do we. Returning to your why—or refining it—is so important. The more you go through this process, the more capacity and resilience builds inside of you for the journey ahead.

There are many different ways for you to discover your why. I suggest starting by writing it down. Create the image in your mind of an identity that you want to embrace. Write it down on paper and then begin to meditate with this image in your thoughts. Ask yourself: *What do I want?* We are often so focused on what we *don't* want that we fail to think about what we *do* want. We don't visualize the bigger picture. We forget to allow ourselves to dream about what our lives could be. Once you decide on what you want and why you want it, start journaling about this version of yourself. You can ask yourself questions like: *What attributes would this person have? How does this person feel emotionally? How do they feel in their body? How are they connected to something spiritually?*

Continue to envision this version of yourself while setting a goal to take the steps needed to become this person. Really dig deep. Do the internal work in order to see this vision as a possibility for yourself. I often hear people say, "I want to lose ten pounds." I prompt them, asking: *When you're ten pounds down, what will you feel like? At ten pounds down, have you really changed anything internally? Have you shifted your mindset? Is it just about the weight?* I find that it's rare for a woman to become a better version of herself by just losing weight. The work is deeper than that.

Instead of making a goal like losing ten pounds, I encourage people to dig deeper on their desires. If you lose ten pounds, it's likely you'll have more energy, you'll have more fun interacting with your kids, and you'll feel grateful for the hard work you've put in. For me, this was a crucial piece. I couldn't just visualize a smaller body. I'd lost weight before without changing my life for the better. I needed to visualize myself feeling happy about parenting, not resentful. I wanted to have huge amounts of energy so that I could go to the park and play rather than sit on the nearby bench feeling irritable. After so many years of feeling doubtful and unworthy, I wanted to have peace. These were the visions that kept me going when being thinner no longer mattered to me.

Sometimes when I hear that a woman has set a goal to "get healthy," it concerns me. Being "healthy" is so nuanced. Each person has a different definition of health. Without putting the right thoughts into this goal, women wind up just adopting someone else's plan for health. Before they know it, they are following a plan that has them working out twice a day and cutting out all of their favorite foods. This often leads to stress, followed by shame and guilt when they're not able to keep up with the standard they've set for themselves. This is often because they didn't have a strong why. When you find your reason why and really work on what that means to you specifically, you set goals based on your personal needs. For example, maybe being healthy means getting eight hours of sleep at night and eating foods that have more sustenance rather than getting minimal sleep and eating foods that leave you feeling sluggish and depleted. Maybe being healthy means you focus on what would fuel your body. Maybe it means focusing on how you can be grateful for your mind, body and soul. From this place, you treat yourself better for the sheer value of doing so.

If there's any hesitation about meeting your goal, you must get back to the basics. Go back to your journal and see if your why is strong enough. Ask yourself: *Are you willing to do whatever it takes to meet your goals?* If there's doubt, keep exploring until you fully understand why it is that you are choosing this path. You must address and explore the psychological reasons you want to change. This is such a valuable process, because a lot of times we may find that our goals are not even our own goals.

They may be part of societal norms, environmental conditioning or we have taken on the rules of someone else's life. For example, maybe it is ingrained in you from childhood that you have to finish everything on your plate. The voice in your head drives your habits, so every time you sit down to eat, you cannot figure out why you're eating more than you need. Are you still holding onto a habit from someone else's value system?

The next step, after visualizing yourself feeling and looking the way you desire is to predict some obstacles. Obstacles are part of life. With anything worth changing, you will experience some resistance, because it matters. Ask yourself: *What will you face that might stop you from achieving this goal? Have you ever been able to accomplish something like this in the past? What are some of the blocks that will prevent you from reaching your goal? What support do you need to reach this goal and do you have those systems in place?*

While there are some physical obstacles, like work schedule or childcare issues, most of our obstacles are faulty belief systems. Thoughts are energy; they play into our emotional exchange. Our emotions are an indicator and predictor of what we will see play out in the physical world. Emotions turn into language, and our language solidifies beliefs and performance. What if you have been hindering your results by the way that you think? Believe me: our belief systems can hurt us. For me, it's interesting to look back on the way I felt that other people viewed me during my youth. It's likely that people didn't view me the way that I thought they did. Instead, I projected onto everyone how I felt about myself (negatively), and from that place, I conditioned my environment to agree with me. When you discover something like this, it's a huge revelation.

Another example in my life is that I held onto the belief that I was failing as a mom, that I just didn't have what it took. I was stuck in such a negative loop that I had little energy for anything more than what I was already doing. My self-worth was low, and all the attempts that I'd ever made to change my body and nutrition had been shame-based. I was coming from a place of fear, which sucked the energy out of me. From this place, fear is all that showed up in my physical world. My thoughts shaped my life and how I felt about it. Staying hyper-focused on failure zapped my energy and overwhelmed me further. Before I knew it, my biggest fears were how I was showing up in my life. What this thinking pattern stole from me was my ability to find beauty and awe in the present moments. Sure, discomfort can exist in those moments, but so does beauty and gratitude and love. You are not your thoughts, and you do not have to become every thought you have.

These same thought patterns can come up when we focus on anything important. Some common faulty beliefs are fear of judgment, perfectionism and distraction. With fear of judgment, you don't want to try and then fail, so you never even start. You might be worried that the people around you will judge you for your failures. Or you might even fear that they will judge you for wanting to change to begin with, for wanting more out of your life. Fear of judgment often results in a person worrying more about what others think of them than what they think of themselves. This cycle can be paralyzing when working toward goals.

I can understand this fear. Maybe it came from being in an environment that was critical and held a lot of judgement. We tend to "wall off" to protect ourselves. But what ends up happening when we hold on to those protective patterns is that we do not evolve past what has happened to us. This can affect our lives and our relationships with self and others in a really negative way. Truth be told, there is no real change without failing and being vulnerable. We have to find a way to cultivate a relationship with ourselves where we silence the inner critic first and take steps with true bravery. We have to get familiar with this process, and with using this failure as feedback to grow and become better versions of ourselves.

Maybe your faulty belief system includes perfectionism. A perfectionist mindset can be a barrier because it's an impossible standard to uphold. During my healing process, I once heard that perfection is a really low standard for yourself. This is so true, because the reality is that you will forever be chasing an unattainable illusion. It can drive you mad and paralyze you at your starting point altogether. People with perfectionism are often held back because they can't start to begin with. They feel like *if I can't do this perfectly, then I'll just wait until I can.* Or they will start, but as soon as something imperfect happens (and it will), they will lose the willpower and stamina to carry on. Unfortunately for perfectionists, the time when everything falls into place and they will be able to flawlessly work on their goals is never going to come. Perfectionism prevents people from starting, and it also is one of the reasons that people give up working on their goals. When they discover that they can't charge toward their goals perfectly by never making mistakes, having slip-ups or facing challenges, they give up. It's too exhausting to go at that pace.

Instead, what we need to learn here is that consistency is the true currency of life and long-term success. Have you heard the quote *"You can never beat the woman who never gives up"*? It is so true. It doesn't matter how perfect you are but rather, how you embrace change and failure. What matters is that you keep going after failure, and in the next moment, shift a little and learn from that imperfection. Aim to get slightly better from each setback. It is consistency in life that breeds intensity. True beauty comes from knowing ourselves and working toward mastery. This is where who we truly are emerges and grows.

Your belief system could also be inhibited because of distraction. Distraction can cause challenges because it easily persuades you to give up on your goals. I used to love a good crash diet. I could get results quickly. For me, crash diets meant giving up on making long-term progress and instead, going for that quick fix. Many people start out with the best of intentions but don't plan for distraction. The minute they feel like progress is stalled or that things aren't moving fast enough, they forsake their goal.

It's easy to be persuaded by the new shiny diet of the month and give up on slow, consistent progress in order to get it over with more quickly. But distractions usually don't last in the long term. What ends up happening is that the distraction leaves us in this perpetual state of chasing. We chase the next distraction. It's like when you are playing a racecar video game, you over-correct and end up swerving all over the road. Big swings one way or the other are really not manageable in the long term. It's the small shifts over time that become habits and leave us more balanced on the road or in life.

I've held all of these faulty beliefs at one time or another, and those beliefs created my reality. In the past, when my goal was to lose weight, I never determined my why or checked in with my mindset. I'd jump on the bandwagon diet of the moment without putting any thought into the emotional side of things. Sure, I had lost the weight before, but it never stuck. I always hit roadblocks, most of which were in my mind. I didn't trust myself to achieve lifelong, sustainable change because I had no experience with something like that. I think deep down, I thought that I didn't deserve to feel good—and therefore sabotaged any progress I made. I didn't have good boundaries, and I'd let other people derail me from my goals. My belief systems around perfectionism, fear of judgment and distraction were holding me back.

Think of yourself as an air filter: all of your priorities are connected. If something is off anywhere in the filtration system, you'll start to have air that's not clear or fresh. Often, when we start overeating or don't want to go to the gym, we think it's *our* problem when in reality, something else is off somewhere. A negative loop is blocking the filter from working properly. I had to learn to find where I should change the filter so I could get clean air running again.

Maybe you're a perfectionist or you fear failure, and you quit the first time you're not able to meet the expectation. Or maybe you're distracted by too many worries. Back when I was experiencing PPD, one of my biggest blocks was that I wasn't shaping up to be the mom I wanted to be. I was so overwhelmed by motherhood and the fact that I wasn't fitting into my idea of what motherhood was supposed to be. I got stuck in my head thinking about what being a *good mom* meant. My air filter was blocked. There was no clean air. This led to poor food choices, numbing and a lack of motivation for change.

Discovering the real reason why you make certain choices or engage in certain behaviors is going to be the true recipe for long sustainable behavior change. In other words, getting clear about your goals and clearing your air filter. This is the key to ensuring that you are not just hopping on the next crash diet or sabotaging your success. It is also key to find the root causes of why we do the things that we do. I was surprised to discover that nutrition was not my real problem at all. It was just the symptom of something greater. My lack of self-worth and belief that I could not take care of myself and love myself properly were the real problems. When you do not believe you are worth it, you will be derailed from your hopes and dreams every time. When you know your worth, you will go to any length to take care of yourself. From that place, you show up for a life of meaning and impact.

I once heard a statistic that 80 percent of the things we worry about happening never actually happen[iv]. This is a lot of wasted energy. Your brain does not differentiate hypothetical situations from real situations. When you have fear, your brain and body react as if something is actually happening to you. Where could that energy be better spent? Instead of worrying about whether or not the change you desire will take place, can you just use that energy to take the next step needed that aligns with your goal? Can you replace that wasted time and energy on things like eating something nutritious, going for a walk, giving yourself grace and saying positive things to yourself?

Once you've established your goal, identified your why, predicted some barriers and roadblocks and worked on your mindset, you might still find that there are challenges. When I'm helping my clients within this structure, I help them identify six categories that are foundational pieces to our lives. These are things that pretty much everybody's working on. You can't work on all six at once because it would be impossible to do well in every category all the time. The categories are career, family, relationships, wealth, physical health and spirituality. If you tried working on all of them at once, you could burn out and become overwhelmed.

You must choose what's most important to you in different seasons of your life. Give a few of those areas your all while allowing others to fall to the wayside for a season. For example, it's going to be very hard for you to work on your physical health if you're going through a tough divorce or a stressful breakup. You might need to focus on working through your grief before you focus on physical health.

When it comes to physical health during a hard season, perhaps you can focus on picking two to three things you can continue to do to take care of yourself. For example, can you hydrate? Can you move, even if it is for a walk? Can you get enough sleep? Maybe you can add nourishing foods, too. Taking care of ourselves in these seasons, in whatever capacity, is so important. Sometimes this self-care might just be what I like to call your "bare ass minimums."

I like to tell this story about when I was in the fifth grade. We were learning how to write research papers. We would go to the library with our notebooks and learn how to take notes and find important information. I always wanted mine to be perfect. I pulled out all the books that I thought I would need (this was long before Google or AI), and used the copy machine to copy the right pages. Then, I learned to take those copied pages and highlight the most important points. Rather than choosing exactly what I would write about however, I highlighted every single word on each page. Soon, my teacher was looking over my shoulder at my highlighted pages.

"Emily, you're going to have to choose what's important," she said. "Not all of this can be in your research paper."

I remember my mind being blown. I thought to myself, *how was I going to decipher what was important?* It was *all* important to me. How was I going to choose where to take a stand and land on a single point? What if I missed something? This was a valuable lesson for me, that not everything can come with you at once. You will have to pick and choose in life where you put your energy and why. This might change depending on you and your season. If you give whatever it is all of your energy and show up genuinely, nothing is ever wasted.

When I was in the position of wanting change in all six categories, I chose physical health and family first. I let all other things go. My career, spirituality, wealth and relationships were not my top priority at the moment. I had to work out these more important things first. That doesn't mean that I didn't come back to those other categories, it just meant that they weren't the most critical at the time.

I needed to get clear about my vision. I created a vision board with a picture of me when I was happy. I cut out words and phrases and added it to my vision board. I journaled about who I wanted to become and the goals I had to meet to get me there. I focused on my why, which was being a happy and energetic mom who could move through depression and sad emotions in a healthy way. I wanted to learn how to be vulnerable and express my grief so that I could see life as beautiful again. I pasted pictures and affirmations on my mirrors.

I made a commitment to stop comparing myself to others, or at least to return to who I was and why I mattered whenever this tendency reared its head. I had an affirmation on my vision board that said: "*Do not compare your Day One to someone else's Day 500. …just keep going.*" This helped me stay out of my head. Whenever I started to feel like I was so far behind, I would return to this phrase and remind myself of my why. I found comfort in the fact that everyone has a "Day One." Change is a process for all of us. I needed to remember that sometimes we see the highlight reels of someone else's life, and not the effort to change not everything that went into it. I wanted things to be different this time.

This time around, working on my mindset was the biggest piece of the puzzle. I used this phrase: "*go slow to go fast.*" In the past, I would change everything all at once. I would start working out every single day, cut calories as much as I could, live a super-restrictive lifestyle for however many weeks. Eventually I'd be so exhausted with it all that I'd just give up the same way that I started. Everything I was doing was so unstable.

This time I had to go slow.

There wasn't just one thing I was trying to change. I wasn't trying to just tweak my diet anymore. I was extremely depressed, I was eighty pounds overweight, I was lethargic and apathetic, and I was lost. I wanted everything to change. When everything needs to change, there's no crash diet to count on. I had to learn to do one thing at a time. True change happens in how you think about things, how you identify with yourself, how you show up day after day slowly over time.

When I couldn't find the internal motivation to keep going, I would look for inspiration. I would read stories of people who'd done what I wanted to do. I found stories of women who came back from pregnancy strong, healthy and with a positive outlook on life.

I looked in my daily life, too. There was a woman in my gym who had previously been living the same lifestyle as I had been. She and I would both tackle the trendiest yo-yo diet. We'd lose a little weight and start feeling good. Then, just as quickly as we started, we'd begin to lose steam and gain weight back. Later on, she got pregnant and I watched her go through the process of having a baby and figuring out her new life as a mom. At the time, she was the only person in our gym to have a baby and then return to work on her physical health. I watched her closely and learned that she was diligent with her diet and her movement. I noticed that she took good care of herself even when she was juggling so much. Soon, she started looking better than she did before the baby and I could see this energy and vitality in her that wasn't there before.

Before seeing her do this, most of the conversations around weight loss and muscle building after pregnancy led me to believe that being healthy, strong and energetic was nearly impossible. Watching her broke through those barriers for me. That was the first time that my mind was opened to the fact that a mom can take care of herself (physically and emotionally) *and* take care of her children. I started to think things like: *what if I could be that diligent and that consistent?* Because of her, I started to build belief in myself about what was possible. I think that humanity thrives off seeing what is possible. We need examples of people who have gone before us.

Finally, it's important to recognize that when someone is facing such a drastic change, it is a deeply personal journey. When I talk about this with my clients, we discuss that it's not just the tug of war *inside* of you but also, possibly, the tug of war *around* you. Maybe some of the people you surround yourself with are not supporting you or they are reflecting back to you things that you don't like about yourself. These can both lead to poor decision-making. In order to make the change you want to see in your life, you might have to change your environment. If there are people in your life not supporting you, you might need to take a hard look to see if these are people you want in your inner circle.

Sometimes the people who don't support you are living with you and you cannot remove yourself from them. If this is the case, you'll need to first understand why this is so important for you (going back to understanding your why). Then, you may have to sit down and have a conversation with them about how you need support. If you're trying to make big life changes and they truly love you, you might have to lead by example. This is true especially if the people in your life have never witnessed this side of you.

Let's talk about how to ask for support from the people that you truly love. First, try writing a letter to get all your thoughts out on paper. This will help you both clarify exactly what you want to say, and help you practice asking for support. Keep in mind that your desired goal might feel unfamiliar and scary to them as well. This is okay. These conversations might need to happen more than once, especially as you get further along in your journey and can better process where you are. Change is something that everyone needs to process in their own time. I have found if you keep showing up with who you want to be , those closest to you will embrace the powerful frame you're standing in. You may be surprised that over time, the powerful impact of your journey can inspire people in your life to take action in their own.

Some say that the five people that we spend most of our time with have the biggest influence on our lives. I urge people to ask themselves a really tough question regarding people who are unsupportive: *Does this person have a place in my life anymore?* Sometimes, removing unsupportive people in your life can make space for those who will support you. It's okay to explore whether you need an environmental shift, and to ask yourself where you can find supportive people who want the same things out of life. It's important to discover how you can build a better support system for yourself. Is it going to a gym? Is it finding a mom's group where you can go for walks while your baby sleeps in the stroller? Is it hiring a coach? Is it finding a free online community? Is it following online influencers who are talking about the goals that you have? There's a saying "energy goes where the attention flows." Sometimes, if the energy in your current situation is negative or unsupportive, you may need to uplevel your environment to get the support that you need to make life-long change.

Working on your mindset from the start of your goal setting

will pay off. It will help you have a more stable and personalized plan. It will help you identify the most compelling reasons for wanting to change. And it will help you to discover why you may have had previous failed attempts or false starts. You'll have more success if you really understand and identify your goals—and the barriers to meeting them. Planning and prediction are pillars of success.

Takeaways

- Lean into the motto *"go slow to go fast,"* which might mean turning away from social media, ads and influencers who are promising a "quick fix."
- Determine your why. Pick something that is compelling and motivating.
- Journal, visualize and create the identity that you want to embrace.
- Determine what the blocks may be. Have you engaged in self sabotage in the past? Are your barriers related to mindset like perfectionism or fear of failure, or are you distracted by something shiny?
- Work through those blocks by digging deep to see why they are there in the first place.
- Create a vision board and use inspiring affirmations that will help you on days when you just don't have the motivation.
- Find people who've gone before you. Lean on them when you lack inspiration for yourself.
- Create a supportive environment and have a heart-to-heart with your loved ones about the deeply personal journey you're planning to go on.

7 FOUNDATIONS OF NUTRITION, PLANNING IS CRUCIAL, AND HOW TO COLLECT DATA

WHEN I SET THE GOAL OF CHANGING MY LIFE, IMPROVING MY nutrition was a major component of this goal. It was the number one thing I wanted to change. I understood that if I properly nourished every system in my body, I could improve my overall foundational health. It was all connected. My body was severely undernourished from my years of dieting/restriction and relying on processed foods when I did eat. In order to work on my depression, my brain and other organs needed vitamins and minerals. I was starting from scratch. I had to learn about how nutrition worked and find the foods that would provide my body with the healthy fuel that it needed to function more optimally.

I couldn't do this alone. I needed help in order to get an understanding of even the most basic things, like what to eat and when to eat it.

I found a coach in my area who was writing nutritional plans for clients, and I hired her. I didn't know what I was doing and I needed direction. I was already so overwhelmed with parenting and my current condition with PPD that I needed my plan to be simple and repeatable. I needed to know what to get from the grocery store, when to eat, how to prepare the food and how to keep going. Another huge part of hiring a coach was to help me set small goals that I could easily achieve. It was helpful to me to have someone remind me to keep going no matter what the day looked like. This was the time I learned the power of consistency. I learned that I have the ability to do hard things and to just keep going.

My coach gave me a nutrition plan that showed me how much protein I was supposed to eat, along with a shopping list and recipes for the week. Because I had worked on my mindset, I was still taking the "*go slow to go fast*" mantra very seriously. I learned which proteins I liked and even how to prepare them. I learned to answer basic questions like: *was it chicken I really wanted or shrimp? How often should I eat red meat and pork? What amount would work for me to feel satiated but still lose weight?*

There's a great quote by Benjamin Franklin that explains my early success. He said "*If you fail to plan, you are planning to fail.*" Planning is crucial when it comes to nutrition. It's not only important to have a vision for your mindset; it's also important to meet your goals around nutrition. I love to make a vision board, and I have done one with my childhood friend many years in a row. Vision planning in community with others can be motivating and inspiring because you speak out loud your goals and wishes for your future self. For the last two years I've made a vision board, everything on it has come true (and for the ones that didn't come true, it is either still in progress or what I wanted shifted into something totally different altogether). There's something really powerful about planning. My friend and I use magazines and other materials to make our vision boards. We use book pages, picture albums and pre-cut words and phrases to make affirmations and mantras. You can use any other materials that speak to you.

If you read good self-help books or listen to podcasts that recommend change, they all start with planning. They may use different strategies or methods, but in all these resources, there is no doubt that planning ahead is a useful tool.

The truth that will change your life is sometimes so obvious that it might feel irritating. Planning might be the hardest thing to do because it's so basic that most people think they understand how to do it. Often, people skip over the planning step or overcomplicate it. In fact, overcomplication can actually be a distraction. You can spend all of your time planning what you are going to do and then never take action.

I help clients focus on the concept that structure equals freedom, not the other way around. No matter who you are, you have to have some parameters in which you operate or things in your life will start to derail. Goals will start to get away from you if you don't have a plan in place and a strong understanding of where you're going. Planning is also a fantastic way to be able to reflect on both what worked and what needs improvement as you keep going. This helps make it okay if a plan changes.

One way I like to frame planning for clients is helping them develop something I call "standard operating procedures" for your life. These are routines that you follow with non-negotiable "bumpers," parameters you don't go outside of. Companies use Standard Operating Procedures to make goals, follow a plan and have success in the workplace. When I adopted this phrase, it was a revelation to me. You have to monitor your bank account if you want to save money. Why would I not do the same thing with my life to be successful with my nutrition, workout routine or other ways that I want to show up for myself?

Not having a plan is also a plan. We are all on a diet, drinking water and walking each day. These are things we do naturally. If you eat food at all, you are on a diet. But an intentional plan for success is something entirely different.

The things you say about yourself and how you define yourself are generally what you will become. For example, if you call yourself a "hot mess," then you will likely act out "hot mess" behaviors. This might mean always being late, taking impulsive actions when it comes to food or showing up in life without intention. That is still a plan, one that your brain is following because it is what you believe about yourself. When I was struggling with PPD and body weight issues, my plan was to numb. I numbed myself with food. I numbed by disconnecting from my loved ones. I planned to only survive the day and counted down the minutes until my babies would sleep.

I often think of people who have hit a rock bottom and need some kind of intervention. Generally, the first part of their recovery is to get on a plan and start following it (like a 12-step program). The same happens when you are trying to make any big change. When I needed help to change my life, making a plan was crucial.

When clients ask me how to begin making their plan, I ask them to really focus on the non-negotiables. What are the things that you will not sacrifice no matter what is going on in your life? Maybe it's getting proper sleep, maybe it's not eating fast food. Maybe it's getting steps in or continuing to set boundaries with that toxic person in your life. Maybe it is about setting boundaries with yourself and keeping your own promises. It's important to start with these, because there will be a time when these things are not easy. There will be seasons of life where survival is necessary–if a family member is sick, or you experience loss of a loved one, or like, me when your babies just won't sleep through the night and you're barely functioning.

What are the non-negotiables that will help you through this season? For example, if you are suffering from exhaustion and your non-negotiable is getting your steps in no matter what, you will still be making progress toward your overarching goals. I've worked with so many clients who—after experiencing a really hard season in their lives—come out on the other side and see that they still made progress by sticking with their non-negotiables. Taking care of yourself in really hard times is the best possible thing you can do for yourself. Difficult seasons are not the time to give up. These seasons are actually the time to lean in and give yourself the love that you need. Let the emotions flow through you as they may need to. From this place, you can truly honor whatever it is you need.

Before planning, when life hit me, I would completely give up on any progress I had made. I wouldn't stick to non-negotiables, and I wouldn't continue to do the things that I needed to properly care for myself. I had a victim mentality. It would sound something like this in my mind: *This always happens to me...why even try.....I can't catch a break. Why can't I be like normal people?* What is normal, anyway? Life happens to us all. This kind of pity party will only slow us down and zap our strength.

I believed that taking care of myself was just one more hard thing that I couldn't do. But I've finally come to understand the beauty and the benefit of coming back to my vision and my plan. No matter what is going on in my life, I tell myself *I'm still the person who wakes my kids up with a smile on my face* (one of my non-negotiables). *I'm still the person who drinks water. I'm still the person who gets my steps in.* I said this all to myself even when I didn't believe it. These non-negotiables become a part of who you are. Before you know it, you're not thinking of them as things you have to get done in a day. They become so routine and so ingrained that they begin to feel as simple as brushing your teeth. It is through doing these things that your identity is formed. When this season passes, your confidence in who you are and what you need will have been cultivated. With each hard moment, your resilience is forged. This is something that no one can take away from you. You become!

This doesn't mean that things aren't hard for me or that I don't ever experience pain. It does mean that I can come back to myself. Instead of trying to control the things that are out of my control—like illness, conflict or kids' needs— I focus on what I can control. What I can control are my reactions and responses to life's current pressures.

You might be wondering how you find your non-negotiables to start with. I encourage my clients to take a very honest look at their lives. What are things that are working for you? What things are not? Go back over the six foundations that I mentioned in Chapter 6 (family, relationships, physical health, spirituality, wealth and career). Which of those areas need the most attention? Which of those areas are going well? Take inventory of the roles that you are playing in your life and make sure that they work for you, not only for everyone else. This might mean answering these questions: *Do I believe I deserve this? Am I valuable enough to show up for myself in this way? Can I offer myself love and forgiveness versus. harsh criticism and judgment? Do I view feedback as failure or an opportunity to grow?*

For example, if your career is very stressful and leaves you with no time or energy, are there things that you can change about that? Do you need to have a hard stop at work so that you have time to cook dinner at home instead of eating out? Find a non-negotiable there like, *I will stop working by 5pm so I can make dinner every night,* and then make it part of your standard operating procedure.

Making a plan might mean learning a new skill or skills. This can often cause overwhelm or fatigue. The more we practice our new skill and make it a part of SOP (standard operating procedure), the easier and more natural it will become. I urge clients to wait at least two weeks (if not more) before changing their plan or giving up on it. It takes time to see if something is working or not, and we don't want to get caught in a trap of constantly changing things based on the emotions of one day or just a snapshot in the bigger picture. We have to give our plan time to gain traction.

I've clarified how important it is to make a plan. Next are some steps that a person can take in order to make a plan specifically for their nutrition. First, if a person wants to lose weight or gain muscle as part of their nutrition plan, they need to determine how much protein, fats and carbs their body needs to function optimally. Proteins, fats and carbohydrates are called macronutrients because they are the three basic foundational nutrients that our bodies must have in order to survive. In other words, they need a balanced diet. A balanced diet usually consists of 30 percent protein, 30 percent fat and 40 percent carbs. This is on average where people start. Every person is different, so this may change after monitoring individual data.

Protein is vital for the body to function optimally. Proteins are made up of chemical building blocks called amino acids. Amino acids are part of all bodily functions including the brain, heart, lungs, hormones and more. Protein is also responsible for building and repairing our muscles and bones. Healthy proteins include, but are not limited to, wild-caught fish and seafood, organic pasture raised beef, pork, bison and organic chicken.

Fat is a vital building block and source of energy in the body. Fats help our bodies absorb certain vitamins and minerals for healthy hair, strong nails and good joint health. Some healthy fats include, but are not limited to, fish oils, egg yolks, nuts and seeds, cold pressed oils, avocado, coconut oil, olives and fat from animal protein. It's a common practice in our society to avoid fats, but it is important to incorporate them into your diet in healthy amounts. They are necessary for the body to function and for hormonal health as well.

Carbohydrates are what give us energy. They are the quick burning fuel that our bodies need to function. Sometimes people refer to carbohydrates as the gas in your fuel tank. Examples of carbohydrates are vegetables, fruits and foods with fiber (which helps our digestive tract), as well as starchy carbohydrates which include things like grains and wheat products.

The best way to look at your diet is that you need a little bit of each of these macronutrients at every meal. If you have a balanced diet of protein, carbs and fat, you will feel satiated. Being satiated for at least 3-5 hours before your next meal is ideal for blood sugar regulation. It is also a good window for your body to do what is necessary to break down food in the digestive tract and transport vital nutrients where they need to go. If you overindulge at one sitting, or if you undereat and are not getting enough nutrients, you are causing imbalance, and this can really stress your body out. Our bodies love balance and to know what to expect on a consistent basis. With this balance, you won't have as many sugar cravings, your mood will be uplifted and you'll have more mental clarity.

Understanding how to eat macronutrients can be life changing, but getting there can feel overwhelming. As with any new skill, it can be challenging at first but becomes second nature with repetition. When you put some skills on autopilot, what once seemed overwhelming is now effortless, and it frees up your mental bandwidth to be able to focus on more.

To learn more about nutrition, it can be helpful to read books or blogs, listen to podcasts or find online education about it. As you get further along in your journey, finding a coach or consultant who can speak directly to you and can take into account your personal traits and other specific important details will help make your plan more clear and effective. I highly encourage finding a specialized plan for this part of your journey. Everyone is different, and working with a coach allows you to understand your body on an individual basis. In addition, your preferences differ from someone else's. You need to understand what works best for you. In addition, the things that you prefer will help you stick to your plan for long periods of time. For example, if you think eating tilapia is what you're supposed to do but you don't like this type of fish, you won't stick with this plan for very long. Some people love more fat and less carbs, and their bodies respond very well to this. They can still reach their goals. The only way to truly know what is working is to track this data with a coach and make small changes over time.

Once you've gotten the right data for your food intake (how much protein, carbs and fat that you need daily), you will need to make a plan for what you will eat. I encourage my clients to find out what staple ingredients they will need to buy at the grocery that have protein, fats and carbs. You need staple ingredients, or meals you like to eat on a consistent basis. This makes the process much easier, trackable and predictable in nature. It also reduces overwhelm and allows you to be more flexible here and there, as you know what the majority of your food day will look like in advance.

I like to tell people to start with foods that they already like. So, for example, if you like chicken, brown rice and broccoli, make sure that you stock up on all of those ingredients. You can cook the chicken, broccoli and rice and have it all ready in the refrigerator. You don't have to make your entire meal ahead of time. Instead, plan ahead so that you have what you need ready to go in the fridge, prepped so you can put together a meal in minutes. Simple, whole food ingredients that have already been prepped can get you from the fridge to your plate in no time.

This is also an excellent way to make sure you can feed your whole family. For example, my kids like tacos, but maybe I don't want tacos for whatever reason. If I already have cooked ground turkey, steamed rice and veggies prepared, I can make the kids tacos and make myself a bowl with very little effort or stress. Meal planning begins by having the right macronutrients simply prepared in order to be able to put together a few meals quickly. Being proactive in these ways will reduce stress and allow for more freedom and flexibility later when you really need it. Planning ahead will keep you from being reactive and feeling like you are always chasing your tail, especially in busy seasons.

When you think of a balanced plate, envision that fifty percent of your plate will be filled with vegetables (like leafy greens, bok choy, cauliflower, brussel sprouts). Next, the plate will have a ½ cup of starchy carbs like sweet potato, pumpkin, beets or carrots. Next, your plate will need 4-6 oz of protein (roughly palm sized). This will be things like chicken, lean turkey, lean organic ground beef or fresh fish. Your plate will need a small amount of healthy fats like nuts, seeds, olives, avocado, coconut oils or ghee. Finally, your plate should have ½ cup whole grains like quinoa, barley or oatmeal.

If you want to go beyond just getting the right nutrients and begin losing weight and building muscle, you will need to find something called your 500 calorie deficit. Losing weight is different from building muscle mass. You will need to be in a 500 calorie deficit in order to lose body fat and hang onto the muscle you already have. This is where the averages and customization will come into play. These will help track how much you are currently eating which sustains your current weight and where your macros will need to be to start losing weight.

Here's what I mean by this: Maintenance calories are the amount of calories that you eat each day when you are not losing or gaining weight. If you want to lose weight you, will need to subtract 500 calories from your current maintenance calories. You will then need to break down the amount of calories that are in fat, protein and carbohydrates. This will give you something called a Macro Count. For example, if your maintenance calories are at 2000 calories daily, and you subtract 500, you get 1500. You now know that you need to eat 1500 calories a day in order to lose weight and build muscle. But this doesn't mean eating 1500 calories of any food. It's likely that you don't just want to lose weight, but also keep it off with a balanced diet full of nutrients that make your body and brain strong. Therefore, you need to make sure that the calories that you do consume have the right amount of protein, carbs and fat. This is what we call "weight loss macros." You can find this breakdown using the image below to do some math to determine exactly how many grams of each macronutrient you need to make up those 1500 calories.

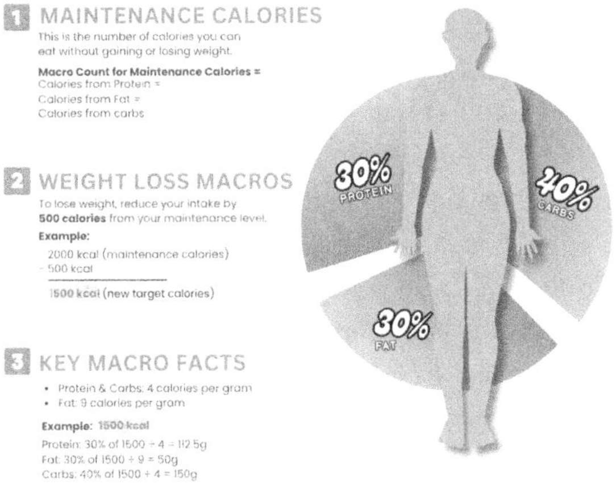

Once you've got the number of macronutrients that you'll eat every day, you will need to start tracking your food. Tracking food means not only logging the foods that you eat each day, but also determining how many grams of each food you consume. The only way to truly know if you're staying within that 500 calorie deficit is to set some markers for yourself. This means weighing your food on a scale. You're going to need to set targets so you know exactly what you're aiming for. If you are outside of that window, you will likely start to gain weight or just stay where you are. This happens to a lot of clients. They reach a place where they aren't gaining weight, but they aren't losing either. They are just maintaining a point on the scale, maybe one where they don't want to be. Tracking that data is what makes the biggest difference for people. If you're just eyeballing your food and not properly weighing it, it is easy to miss the mark on that 500 calorie deficit. This is why getting a scale, and putting your plate on that scale, is so important. You can measure the exact volume of each ingredient so that you know exactly what you're putting in your mouth. The key is to understand both what foods you are eating and also how much. This doesn't mean you will have to track to this extent forever. It will require some up-front work, though, to know where you are and to make adjustments in order to get to where you need to go.

You want to think of your body like a bank account. If you need to save money for something like a down payment on a house, then you are going to need goals. You need to know what's coming in and what's going out, and you probably need to live below your means to stash away extra money. It's the same with your body. If you want to lose weight and make sure that you're burning fat (and not just quickly lose water weight and muscle tone), you're going to need to know exactly how many calories are coming in from food and going out from exercise.

Usually when I talk about weighing food, people say things like *"I can't go that far"* or *"that seems obsessive."* I get it. I used to think things like *what am I going to do, carry this scale around with me?* But the reason this feels so extreme is because generally, we lack a lot of understanding about food and nutrients. Over the years, fad diets have replaced food education. Instead of learning why a diet actually works, we just follow along with a plan and hope for the best.

I think it's important to understand why fad diets work in general. When you're using something like *Weight Watchers* or Intermittent Fasting, the diets are a tool that hopefully gets you to that 500 calorie deficit. Everybody needs to be in a 500 calorie deficit to lose weight. That is the bottom line when it comes to weight loss success. For example, with *Weight Watchers*, there is a point system, and you must remain at or under a certain number of points to reach your weight loss goals. Intermittent Fasting decreases the window of when you eat so you're more likely to eat fewer calories than it takes to maintain your current weight, and you start to lose weight. If you want to do *Weight Watchers* or Intermittent Fasting, they can be good tools as long as you understand that you have to eat under your metabolic baseline in order to lose fat.

I'd done fad diets, but when I finished them, I still had no understanding of what my body really needed. I needed to track. I had no understanding of how food worked, and I needed to learn this in order to meet my fitness goals. So yes, there were times that I had to carry my scale around! You must use data to track your progress. Do you look over your finances regularly? The answer is yes. If you want to do something big, like save money to buy a house, you have to work at it and you have to do things outside of your comfort zone. You might have to say no to things that everyone else is saying yes to. This is what it takes when you're working on your physical health, too.

There are great apps that can help with tracking. I use *My Fitness Pal,* a health and nutrition app that helps you learn about your food habits, monitor your diet and reach your health goals. It provides you with data that helps you understand the food that you are eating. Without this data, you won't know what led to losing one pound or why you aren't reaching your goal though you did the week before. Most women that I work with know that they need to eat more protein, but without tracking, it is hard for them to get the exact amount their body needs. Using this tool is my top tip for starting out. Data is essential in any weight loss journey.

When I hired a consultant to help me with my nutrition, I learned that I had been using sauces and seasonings on all of my food, which was adding a lot of unnecessary calories. By using a personalized meal plan, I learned different ways to add flavor to my food so that it tasted good, but with fewer added calories or processed ingredients. I used meal planning to help me avoid things like sugar crashes or overeating when I was bored or tired. I had a rule, though: All of my meals had to have five ingredients or less and be ready in 15 minutes. I began eating lean meats, healthy fats and good carbohydrates. I focused on eating more veggies and ate fruit with most of my meals. I even began learning what fast food options would work to fuel my body.

Some of my go-to meals were:

Strawberry Crunch Salad

Ingredients

1 cup cabbage
1 cup spinach
1 handful Trader Joe's EBTB mixed nuts
1 small cucumber
1 small radish
1 cup strawberries
½ cup mozzarella
2 tsp Trader Joe's dill mustard
⅓ avocado
4 oz turkey breast

Directions

Cut, chop, mix and enjoy!

Taco Cups

Ingredients:

12 corn tortillas
2 lbs of ground beef
Shredded cheese
Salsa, guacamole or your favorite taco topping

Directions:

Take a 12-cup cupcake pan and place one corn tortilla in each cup
Saute 2 lbs of ground beef
Put ground beef into each tortilla to make a taco cup

Sprinkle favorite cheese (half a handful or less for all 12 cups)
Bake at 350 for 20 minutes
Top it with salsa, guacamole or whatever you like to eat on your taco

I also ate a lot of homemade "bowls." To me, bowls are a base of healthy carbs topped with veggies and protein that I like. I love Brussels sprouts bowls, with Brussels sprouts as the base, lean meat like chicken or shrimp, finished with cheese.

I was once at a party that was potluck-style. A friend brought something she called "loaded sweet potatoes." I started to play around with her recipe on my own, and I now eat loaded sweet potatoes all the time. Sometimes, I use her original recipe: ground meat of your choice (like beef or turkey) over a medium sweet potato, cooked in the oven at 400 degrees, and topped with cheese, salsa and other veggies when it's done.

The more you learn about proper macronutrients, the more balanced each meal will become. By focusing on macronutrients, you will see benefits in all areas of health. You will find that you are losing weight or maintaining your desired weight. You will have more energy for longer periods of time (instead of short bursts of energy created by blood sugar spikes from foods like baked goods, white flour and pasta). You will have mental clarity and improved sleep. You should also see improvements in your mood.

I could no longer just wing it when it came to the food I consumed. I had to decide what I was going to eat, how much I would eat and when I would eat it. This took work, but the planning helped me become successful and make progress on my goals. Working with someone took a lot of guesswork out of what I needed to do. I had never been successful at anything like this before. I was learning the new skill of how to eat, and I had a plan to support myself. I started gaining more skills and more confidence. Before long, I got really good at creating my own meals.

Proper nutrition and a balanced plate filled with macronutrients is good for hormone health. Whether you're a new mom or someone who is approaching perimenopause or menopause, your diet can be a tool for success through these difficult times of hormone fluctuation. It's important to understand that consuming too much or too little of any one macronutrient can cause a nutritional imbalance. Increasing your protein intake decreases the effects of the hormones that make us hungrier—and increases the levels of the hormones that make us feel full. This stabilizes our blood sugar and supports the maintenance of our bodies. Increased protein also stabilizes our gut health, since serotonin (the hormone that regulates mood) is found in the gut. Having stable gut health helps you absorb more vitamins and nutrients in the rest of your body. The more you eat good food in a balanced manner, the better your body is going to function.

On the most basic level, if there's an imbalance in the way that you eat, then you are going to have an imbalance in your hormones because our food source is the fuel that our body uses in order to function. Maintaining a good balance of food means that your body can use its resources to help balance whatever area needs help. If you're not eating healthy, nourishing food, then your body will use the resources it gets from food to protect your most vital organs like your heart first. It will not support other parts of the body, and the first to let go is the female reproductive system, because those systems aren't vital to staying alive. Over time, having hormone balance can really affect your life in a positive way—and it starts with a good balanced diet.

The next step in learning about nutrition as a foundation for long-term success is understanding hydration. When you're dehydrated, you can feel hungry, which can lead to unnecessary snacking or poor food choices. The signals and sensations in our bodies when we are thirsty are the exact same as hunger signals. Sometimes it's easy to get confused. Proper hydration is the number one thing you can do to support your body overall. Hydration can fight off fatigue and mental fog, and can improve your capacity for better food choices. Sometimes it is good to ask yourself, *am I hungry or thirsty? Should I drink something first and see if my perceived hunger signals subside?* When I started, I had a favorite cup that held 30 ounces of water. I aimed to fill it up at least three times a day.

Being more intentional about how much water you drink can go a long way in meeting your health goals. Typically, we drink less than we need. To get in enough water, we can use the mantra, "go slow to go fast." Increase your water intake by ten or twenty ounces a day. You can find hydration calculators online. These will help you calculate your needed water intake by your weight and your activity level. The suggested standard is .5 ounces for every pound of body weight. Once you discover the ideal amount, just start to gradually increase until you meet your goal.

Another area that can either help improve or actually hinder your nutritional goals is sleep. Lack of sleep can create a lot of stress in your body. The stress it creates usually leads to inflammation. With inflammation, your body starts to retain water and it can greatly affect your ability to lose weight. Lack of sleep is associated with myriad diseases. It is also linked to many chronic health problems including heart disease, kidney disease, high blood pressure, diabetes, stroke, obesity and depression.

If you've ever had a night when you didn't sleep well, you may have found that you craved carbohydrates the next day. This was because you didn't have a lot of energy and carbs are quick burning fuel. Craving carbohydrates is your body's way of telling you *I need energy to do this.*

Not getting enough sleep is also going to affect your readiness to move. Your motivation to exercise or get your steps in will be lower, and continuous lack of sleep can really impact long term goals.

It's not good for the body to do hard workouts on little sleep.

If, for example, the baby kept you up all night, maybe just go for a walk and give yourself the rest that you need. Try to take a nap if you can and focus on doing less around the house or at work. If you're someone who struggles to nap, that is okay. The point I am trying to make is that rest is about truly doing less, keeping your heart rate low and your physical stress to a minimum. Yes, I'm saying to forsake your to-do list for rest! Once you're rested, you can resume your normal workout routine.

One way to help improve sleep is to detach from the environmental disruptors that keep us wired. This can include bright lights, flashing screens and loud noises. Your wind-down routine could start by literally turning down the television and dimming the lights in your home. I would suggest opting for a lamp instead of harsh overhead lighting. Avoid aggressive activities that increase adrenaline. Minimize screen time and/or use blue light blocking glasses. Find an activity to do before bed that is calming like reading, listening to meditative music or listening to a relaxing podcast. Foster an environment that is soothing, just as you would for a baby who you want to sleep through the night. Allow that natural rhythm to take shape.

When it comes to building a solid foundation for your nutrition, there are many steps that, if taken seriously, will have a huge impact on results.

Takeaways

- Make a plan and take it seriously. Develop your Standard Operating Procedures.
- Determine your non-negotiables and stick to those at all times. Especially during difficult seasons.
- Hire a coach, or get personalized help on the basics of what foods your body needs to be successful.
- Begin tracking your food / weighing your food to collect data and ensure that you are meeting your

nutritional needs (use an app like *My Fitness Pal*). Extra focus on macronutrients (protein, carbs and fat).
- Properly hydrate and track that progress as well.
- Promote healthy sleep habits.
- Use a balanced diet of macronutrients to promote hormone health.
- Return to your plan and your why when you feel discouraged or are questioning if your methods are extreme or intense.

8 WHEN YOU FEEL BETTER, YOU DO BETTER: INCORPORATING MOVEMENT

IN THE BEGINNING OF MY JOURNEY, CHANGING THE WAY THAT I ATE and following a meal plan was very hard. I didn't trust myself. Trust is the biggest reason I tell people to hire a coach. Coaching is so much more than just accountability and data tracking with a trained eye. It is a trusting and loving relationship that you build. Your coach can help show you the journey and build your trust in yourself. The biggest thing we can get from the support of others is their belief in us until we can believe in ourselves.

I didn't expect the scale to budge because it hadn't in the past. I did have intense feelings about making sure that I was doing this exactly right. These feelings came from a good place. I wanted to make sure I *did* succeed this time. I had no track record or frame of reference for success, and the amount of weight that I had gained made me feel like I had to be perfect. My perfectionism started to creep back in. I was hard on myself when I had a misstep or when things didn't go perfectly. Later, I would come to realize that my perfectionism was really just self-sabotage. At the time, I was comfortable operating from a place of extreme self criticism and with a perfectionist mentality. I was not yet clear on how this mindset was hindering my efforts. I just didn't understand that consistency was more powerful than perfect.

Not only is it more powerful than perfect, it is the secret sauce that breeds true change in our lives. Consistency is the only thing that can help battle the resistance we experience when something worth doing isn't always easy. When I started my journey, I relied heavily on my meal plan without ever adding any of my own input. This was okay at first because I was so desperate. Sometimes you need to build consistency in your life first, especially when you're at a loss to even know where to start. It helps free mental bandwidth. Later, once you've built some trust with yourself, you can explore what being healthy looks and feels like to you. We all have to start somewhere. The play-by-play from the proverbial (and literal) handbook is a great place to do so.

I can remember when I first realized that I was the heaviest I had ever been. I thought there was a hair that kept brushing up against my back. When I reached back to brush it away, I realized it wasn't hair; it was excess skin from my weight gain. I was shocked. I had never felt fat on my body like that before. The revelation stopped me in my tracks. I thought to myself *how far gone is too far gone? Do I do nothing and keep letting this go? Or do I change?* These were not easy questions to answer. But you are never stuck unless you stop trying.

For me, these questions offered moments of deep truth. I was made for more. I knew that! No one was coming to save me. That is the most daunting and freeing revelation a person can come to in their lives. It is from this place we can actually give ourselves permission to start showing up and truly live. The feelings of guilt and shame were overwhelming. I realized that I had chipped away at my own self-confidence by breaking the biggest promise that I had ever made to myself: that I would stay fit and healthy. Finding this excess skin on my back brought me to my darkest place. My mind kept telling me things like, *you don't actually love yourself* and *you don't care about yourself at all.*

Sitting with this made me very sad. When I felt stressed about learning a new skill while taking care of my new babies, I reminded myself of that feeling. I reminded myself that my babies need a mom who loves herself. I returned to my affirmations like "just keep going." My why was strong enough to get me through those hard and stressful times. My babies were counting on me their lives depended on my healing. I had decided within my soul that I was going to do whatever it took to become who I needed to be for my kids. I wanted them to experience the love that they deserved from me. However, I was well aware I couldn't give to them what didn't already exist within me first.

Part of my plan was to take pictures and measurements of myself, as well as weigh myself, at the beginning of my journey and every four weeks after. It was so basic at first, but existing in these boundaries created a solid foundation that I needed to start. When I stepped on the scale four months after starting my nutrition plan, I saw I had started to lose significant weight. This was so encouraging to me. Nothing will motivate you more than a taste of success. I think celebrating all the small victories along the way motivates us as well. The small victories add up and keep forward momentum going. When I started my journey, I thought that hitting a certain number on the scale or losing a certain amount of weight was going to make me a happier person—that losing weight was the key to happiness. Instead, I found I cared more about becoming a solid, honest human being who did what she said she was going to do. The motivation from sticking with a plan, eating a balanced diet and talking myself through my mental battles brought me to tears. This motivation was weaving all the broken promises and fractured identities inside of me into a thread of truth I could find again. I could be someone that mattered. Not for the world, but for me.

The motivation and the confidence that this built inside of me was astounding! I did what I said I was gonna do. I knew deep down that nobody could take this truth away from me: I am who

I say I am. The confidence that I gained was better than the weight loss. If I could show up like this for my nutrition, what else could I do? The possibilities were endless. There is nothing you cannot do when you know exactly what you want and why. I wanted to keep putting this plan to action. I wondered what other areas could use this same approach.

I thought about a motivational quote, "You can be or do anything you want to be or do." I suddenly wondered if it was true. Up until this point, I didn't think so. I thought that was only true for people out there who were gifted beyond measure. I had no idea that it might apply to me. I love this quote: "You cannot beat the person who never gives up." You just can't! It might not be immediate, but if you don't stop, you can change your life. These quotes are not only for the gifted and talented. They are for the ordinary person just like you or I. They are there to show us what is possible and inspire us to trust our gut instincts. You and I, my friend, were created for more.

Once I saw results on both the scale and in my mental health, I finally had the motivation I needed to keep going. I was gaining so much confidence in myself for sticking with my plan and pushing through hard times. I literally could not believe that I could do this. I couldn't believe that I was this mentally tough. I had started and stopped diets and weight loss tactics so many times in my life that I had lost all trust in myself. But now, I was seeing changes and I wanted to keep going for myself. I wanted to see what more I could accomplish. I was truly moving from doing this because I loved my kids to doing this because I loved and valued myself.

Before this, deep down, I didn't feel like I was worthy enough to show up for myself. As I continued making gains toward my goals, I saw that it was not only okay but *essential* to show up for myself. That's when the real work started to take shape. I was motivated and ready to see how far I could take my goals.

I was ready to move my body again. I went back to the basics and remembered how important being active had been throughout my life. Sports, group fitness classes and going on walks or runs had always been a source of joy. I hadn't moved in two years but now that my body was being properly fueled, I found my way back to the motivation I needed to start moving.

I began my way back to movement by tracking my steps. I decided that I could start by just going for a 10-minute walk while pushing the stroller. I noticed that the more I moved, the more I wanted to move. Over time, that one 10-minute walk turned into two separate 10-minute walks. Looking back, I think this was the perfect way to start. Starting slow in order to gain intensity in my flow, I was ultimately able to move fast as I built my new habits. Why was this the perfect time? Because after having a baby, nothing comes back in a speedy manner. You must give yourself recovery grace. It was the perfect opportunity for me to focus on what I could do each day and just keep it moving.

Then I learned how to do bodyweight exercises and got dumbbells so I could exercise at home as much as my time would allow. This also allowed me to build more confidence. I embraced starting from the ground up and built a new foundation in this way. I tried to incorporate resistance training one day a week with the idea that I could eventually increase both the weight and the number of days I used them. If I started a workout, and 10 minutes in, one of the babies started crying, my mindset was always *at least I got ten minutes in.*

I had to reframe my mindset and think that after being sedentary for so long, any amount of movement was better than none. I also had to reframe my mindset and realize what worked for me before I became a mom might not work for me any more. Maybe, just maybe, I could get curious about what would work for me now and dig deep to develop a new normal. It's said that the most mentally healthy people are adaptable and flexible. This was the foundation of the new skills I was learning. That was my initial non-negotiable.

By going slow, I was building the foundation for new habits. Everyday, I grew stronger and I wanted to work out even more. I knew this would be a challenge without help. I talked with my husband and we agreed that we would hire somebody to help take care of the kids. We hired a nanny so that I could go to the gym. Someone came over a few hours a day, a few times a week, so that I had time to myself. This was a game changer for me. It was the first time I was able to see how a little bit of alone time could energize me and allow me to show up for my kids as well. I was getting the breaks I needed. I was able to be present and enjoy moments with my babies instead of feeling resentful that my whole life had changed.

When I first got help, it didn't feel comfortable. I had mom guilt, which came as a surprise to me. I remember feeling it so powerfully when I started leaving the kids with the nanny to take time for myself. I was torn between taking care of myself and taking care of my kids. What I realized, though, was that I couldn't take care of them from where I stood at that moment. I still had work to do. I needed to care for myself first. Guilt is a liar. But I had to learn to question my guilt. *Just because I'm feeling guilty, does that mean that I actually am? Could these guilt trips we put ourselves in actually be lying to us?* Because in reality, taking care of ourselves and spending time alone is necessary to our mental health.

As I pulled out of the driveway for my first trip to the gym, I wasn't sure if I was making the right decision to leave my babies behind to go work out. Even more, I wondered if I should use that time to get other tasks and errands done. I thought, *Is it a waste to focus solely on working out when I have so much to do?* I had planned for this, though. I knew that this was an old feedback loop playing in my brain. This was the exact moment I began to question the program running in my subconscious. I got in my car, buckled my seatbelt and slowly pulled out of the driveway. I got halfway down the street, turned around and pulled back into the driveway. I was literally driving up and down the street trying to decide if I should go or not.

I finally decided to go. Even though it wasn't easy, I had to learn to put my mental and physical health first. I returned to my why and asked myself important questions about the resistance that I was feeling. I would say things to myself like: *I'm someone's sole caretaker for 24 hours a day. Surely it's okay that I take the two hours I need today to take care of me.* I ultimately decided that it was okay and pulled out of the driveway to go to the place I really needed to be.

When I made it to the gym, I tried doing deadlifts with the weights I'd used many years before. I was sore for days, and I was humbled. I realized that I would have to show up every day, and do a little bit better than the day before. This helped me to be consistent and to allow myself some grace.

Some of the questions that I encourage women to ask when they are faced with resistance or guilt from using their time to exercise are: What keeps me motivated to continue participating? What mental strengths do I possess? Who can I turn to for help? What can I control? What will I gain from exercising right now versus not moving my body?

You want to think about the full picture. If you take care of yourself first, it not only affects you physically but emotionally and spiritually as well. Taking care of yourself means you are showing up for your loved ones for the long game. You want to be there in the best mind and body possible. This means sometimes taking time away from them so that you can take the best possible care of yourself.

As women, we must begin to get comfortable with letting things go. If your choice is to either go for a walk or fold laundry, you should choose the walk. The walk will provide endorphins that your body so desperately needs, and your partner can pick up the household duties. If you have the means, consider joining a gym that offers childcare. If you must do chores, find ways to build in movement. Simple changes like taking the stairs instead of the elevator when possible and parking farther away from entrances when running errands can make a big impact.

Starting a new routine or exercise plan can be overwhelming. I suggest to my clients that they start by finding the easiest and the most basic things to do. For example, do you walk? If you do, can you start to be more intentional with walking? Can you look for 10-minute breaks in your day to clear your mind and go for a walk? Can you do this a couple of times a day? Can you make a date to walk with another mom at the park and push the stroller? Can you find time to do two 10-minute walks to focus on increasing your daily step count? I've found that the easiest way for women to add more activity into their life is to start with walking.

The reason our watches track 10,000 steps a day is because fitness professionals have determined that this number will take a person from a sedentary to an active one. In my coaching program, I encourage women to walk between 8,000 and 10,000 steps a day when starting moving again. If that feels like a lot, I ask them to average 8,000 to 10,000 steps over the course of seven days. That gives them more flexibility.

Once a person gets into the habit of moving 10,000 steps a day, it becomes about stacking habits one at a time. Someone might start by building up to that step count and then over time, increase their workouts to add in strength training. I ask women if they can add some strength training in one day a week, then slowly increase up to three times a week. Building muscle is so important for women, but if you have not done it in a while (or ever), it can feel very daunting. I find it easiest to just start slow and build your intentionality around movement.

One of the most common misconceptions that I hear from women is that they don't want to lift weights because they're afraid that they will become bulky. That's just not true. It takes months, if not years, to gain muscle bulk, and there are so many factors that go into making that happen. Building muscle does not equal muscle bulk. If you pair strength training with the proper nutrition, you can develop whatever type of physique you want.

Building muscle means strength training. This is important for women for different reasons. Many women find that when they start a new diet or workout plan, they end up losing the weight they want but they have a body that looks the same, just smaller. Strength training can help women build the physique that they want. Building muscle is also important for longevity. We sometimes need to think beyond what we want to look like right now to how we want our bodies to feel as we age. Think forward to when you are 80 years old; are there things that you want to be able to do freely?

We need to think about the quality of life we want to have at the end of our lives and start working toward that now. Do you want to walk as best as you can and not use a wheelchair? Do you want to have the most energy you can for engaging socially? Connection is so key to our lives and we suffer without it. Do you want to be able to use your mind and think critically? Think about it this way whatever you don't use, you will most definitely lose over time. The greatest way to safeguard our health and fight off diseases at the very foundation is to continue to build muscle.

Putting muscle on your frame is the key to longevity and having energy later in life. How you age, how well your body is going to move, the vitality of your organs and how they function well into your old age—these are all dependent on having muscles. I encourage women to think about those sweet babies that they've brought into this world—one day those babies are going to have their own sweet babies. If you want to be a grandparent who is able to run around with their grandkids, walk freely without the use of a walker and have a fit mentality and a functioning body, you're going to have to have muscle.

There are many free strength training workouts online. Find one that feels both fun and challenging and add it into your workout routine. Once it starts feeling easy, consider increasing the weights. Maybe you start with body weight, then add ten pound dumbbells, then add twenty pounds or even more as you begin to gain strength. Strength training doesn't have to be hard or complicated, but if you are able to hire help, I suggest hiring a personal trainer in order for you to learn and ensure that you are doing it safely. Over time, you will understand what it takes to strength train and maybe you won't need as much help. Getting help can also provide you with ideas you might need to create a workout plan that is easy for you and fits into your schedule.

In addition to getting steps and building muscle, there are other things that we need to do to help our bodies be strong and fit. Focusing on cardiovascular health is important for better heart health. Stability and mobility work like yoga and stretching ensure that you work your joints through a range of motion to keep them fluid and strong. I want clients to know that what they do now when it comes to physical fitness can improve your quality of life later. For example, let's say you're doing core work and have muscle on your frame. If you fall down the stairs, you'll be better positioned to brace yourself and stop the fall. Or even if you do take a stumble—because we all do—having muscle on our frame prevents extreme injury and can help you in recovery as well. It is so vital. I cannot stress it enough.

To keep things fun and exciting, I like to teach clients to focus on different workouts through different seasons. In winter, for example, it's darker in the mornings and darker in the evenings. It might be hard to get motivated to go out and do a long walk when it's cold and dark. So, maybe winter is a time to focus on strength training. When spring and summer come around and people can be outside more often, they can incorporate hiking, swimming, paddle boarding or whatever else feels fun! Do you like to play tennis or run? Building in activities that require movement but are also fun is a great way to keep your body strong and healthy. If there is anything I have learned along the way, it's that if you hate it, you won't be doing it long, but if you love it, you just won't ever stop. That is the flow we are looking for in our lives. It may come with some trial and error, but get curious about what you need and what you love when it comes to movement.

People tend to think they have to do a lot of cardio in order to lose weight. But what it takes to change your body composition is really quite simple. It's building muscle to burn fat. Technically speaking, our heart rate needs to be 120 or below to build muscle. This is a parasympathetic state, which is a more restful place than if your heart rate is 140 or higher (which is usually where our heart rate is during cardio). A heart rate at 140 or higher burns the carbohydrates left in the body as fuel, so you can burn a meal for that day. Cardio alone is not what changes your composition or gives you the look you desire.

Once you build muscle, you're able to burn calories beyond the time that you're actually exercising. The issue with only doing a bunch of cardio is that you are just burning the carbohydrates in your body. You won't continue to build and develop muscle or burn calories throughout your day. Having more muscle on your body will also allow you to eat more calories. People with more muscle can withstand a higher calorie diet than people just starting out, and who doesn't want more food?

Cardio doesn't build muscle on your frame. It increases your cardiovascular strength and burns what is currently in your system, but it ends when the workout ends. I personally believe that a person needs cardio *and* muscle building to be balanced and healthy. Both are necessary in my opinion, but we typically over-emphasize things like fancy HIIT (high intensity interval training) workouts, races and grinding the cardio wheel alone as a societal norm.

When it comes to movement, it's about understanding and focusing on what moves the needle forward for you instead of focusing on things that are not moving the needle forward. Much like I talked about in other chapters, when it comes to movement, you can't focus on all the things you want to do at once. In fact, I think this is what makes fitness seem so complicated in our society. Instead of trying to focus on everything at once, a person needs to come up with a plan that shows them results and make it part of their regular habit.

My goal became "plan, execute, evaluate." I made a plan, I followed through with the plan, and then I carefully evaluated what was working. If something wasn't working, I changed it and started again. Plan, execute and evaluate. Each time I planned and followed through, my confidence grew and so did my success rate.

Over time, movement became about more than just weight loss and mental clarity. It became a hobby, a source of joy and my favorite form of self-care. One of my favorite moments was when I joined a boutique fitness studio that had childcare. I had fallen in love with a rhythm-based cycling class and I got really good at it. I never missed a class and couldn't wait until the next one. It was also a space for me to interact with other adults and have a social life, which sometimes seemed impossible while parenting two babies.

One day I was at the gym, getting ready to go to my favorite cycling class, and I saw that the studio was looking for a new instructor. I was with my friend, and she encouraged me to apply. I liked the idea of this, but I had to audition, and the whole process made me feel nervous. But because my nutrition was balanced and movement had become so important to me, I finally had the confidence to do something like this. I tried out and was invited to train to become an instructor. I went through rigorous training and even had to pass exams in order to be able to teach my own cycling class, but I did it! I became an instructor. Doing something like this at any earlier point in my life would have been an absolute no-way for me. I lacked the confidence to believe I could be a leader in this part of my life. The moment I gave myself permission to show up for myself, when I pulled out of my driveway and went to the gym, was what paved the road for me to believe in myself. I was made for more and I could now finally be exactly who I wanted to be (even when the previous season of my life had suggested otherwise). It is never too late to reinvent yourself or to go after things that scare you.

Because I was new, I was given a timeslot that no one else wanted—Sunday mornings. I made the most of that time. It went from being a time that was never full to an always-packed house. We called it church because it gave me and the other women (mostly all moms) the time that we needed to get back to ourselves. The room was dark and the music was so good. It felt spiritual at times. We were all going to go back to our lives after class, but in class, we found our souls in the cracks of our to-do lists and roles. It was life-giving. And I was getting stronger with every class. I will always look back at that time and think about how special that room of women was. We were vulnerable with each other in a way where we didn't have to say too much. Our vulnerability is what connected us.

I began to teach more classes and learned that I wanted to get back to teaching. The more I learned through becoming a fitness instructor, the more I wanted to know. I developed a fascination with food and how certain foods fueled us and others depleted us. Since I was already helping people with movement, I wanted to learn more about the nutrition side. I wanted to help people understand that food played an important role in maximizing their level of fitness overall. In the studio that I was teaching in, there was a functional medicine doctor who worked with clients to understand metabolic dysfunction. At times, I worked under her to help support our clients. I loved coaching people through the process of not just what to eat and why, but all the reasons we don't do what we know to be good for us. I became aware that if you can change the programming in your mind, you can change your life. I found myself craving more knowledge and wanting to learn the science behind food and our brains/bodies.

The functional medicine practitioner highly recommended an educational program called Nutritional Therapy. I went through a year-long program, learning the most important foundations of the body including gut health, blood sugar regulation, fatty acid deficiency, hydration, mineral balance and all the other things that keep our body working optimally and out of metabolic dysfunction.

Metabolic dysfunction is what happens when something alters the body's processing and distribution of macronutrients (proteins, fats and carbohydrates). I was starting to understand what metabolic dysfunction was and how it shifts ever so slightly each year just by the way we treat ourselves. For example, when you have metabolic dysfunction, your hormones become imbalanced, and when hormones are imbalanced, it causes inflammation in the body. Inflammation causes diseases and autoimmune issues, and can even lead to cancer. I was fascinated by the crucial roles that food, movement, sleep and water play in how we thrive.

Before gaining this understanding, I didn't know that these things (food, water, sleep, movement) were the foundation of health. I just assumed that you were fine until you got sick. Then, you would go to the doctor or the hospital and they would tell you what you had. I didn't know that there were preventative measures for so many diseases and disorders. I didn't know that it was all connected. The journey to health is so pivotal.

After I went to nutritional therapy school, I was even more passionate about becoming a practitioner. I could help people dial in to what we all can control health-wise, what we put in our mouth and how we treat our body. I helped others find the missing piece. By taking care of my body and mind, I gained so much. There was value that was directly connected to my psychological and emotional state. This trickled down into all aspects of myself. When you feel better, you do better.

If you plan but don't take action, time and time again, you begin to feel like shit. You stop trusting yourself. Your negative thought patterns creep in, and your air filter gets clogged. Every time I planned and executed, I had the opportunity to evaluate the small wins, slow progress and the major epiphanies that were beginning to transform my life. Not only was my body finally reflecting the real me, but my mind was, too. It started so slow, but then it was all at once. I woke up one day and everything was different. *I did that,* I thought. *I made that happen!* Knowing that I was able to make it all happen was exhilarating. Knowing that I now had the skills to handle any major issue that came my way, in a really sustainable way, was invaluable. You become so powerful when you treat yourself as valuably as you are. You deserve to be here, because you are here! Never let any shitty circumstance convince you otherwise.

Takeaways

- Enlist help so that you can carve out enough time to move your body. Hire a babysitter, find a gym with a daycare or swap with other moms.
- Start with the most basic movement and commit to moving every day.
- Educate yourself on why you're moving and what each exercise does for your body, brain and overall health–not just today, but as you age as well.
- Begin to understand the importance of building muscle and start stacking workouts, going from once a week to twice a week.
- Find free resources like *YouTube* videos or websites for basic weight training and buy a set of dumbbells for home workouts.
- Find physical activities that are fun for you. You will feel more motivation to move if you're doing something that you enjoy.

9 ACCOUNTABILITY THROUGH COMMUNITY

My transformation wouldn't have lasted without my community. This sentence alone is probably one of the most crucial points I can make and what I want every reader to get out of this book. When you are in need, you absolutely need a community of support around you. Connection is the key to life. The greatest hindrance in our society is isolation, yet it becomes so normalized. We have these unspoken rules that many of us live by: don't feel too much because it's a sign of weakness, pick yourself up by your bootstraps and be totally independent. The truth is, you are more powerful when you are connected to a community—and more successful when you do it with help.

If you're in a place where you are trying to get somewhere that you have never been—or become somebody you've never seen, or never been able to become—it is very difficult to do it on your own. Sometimes history tells you that it's impossible. What you need to see is the hidden possibility found in each moment and someone else's belief that you can borrow, or even their example of what can be done.

I had come a long way in meeting my goals. My nutrition was balanced and I was on my way to becoming a nutrition coach. My fitness was back to normal and I found that I most enjoyed coaching my fitness classes and teaching other women about health. I was strong and motivated, but I wanted to go further. I could only go so far on my own. Even with all of my background in group fitness and nutrition, I needed help. I still had a relationship with food that I didn't love. It was very emotionally charged when I didn't feel in control. My fitness was sometimes borderline obsessive and I could really beat myself up if I missed a day. I was looking for more freedom and reassurance that perfection is a really low standard for myself. How could I learn to just approach it one day at a time and one season at a time?

I discovered a woman who was working with a community of women regarding nutrition. Her *YouTube* shorts started popping up on my feed and we became friends over social media. I was intrigued by her content because what she was teaching hadn't been an area of focus for me yet. I hadn't yet figured out how to have freedom with food. I understood macronutrients and how to keep my body functioning optimally, but I still used restriction at times. I still considered some foods "bad" and other foods "good."

This would lead to not getting enough nutrients for as long as I could go and then bingeing later. It was becoming a vicious cycle.

Before watching her videos, it hadn't occurred to me that your body breaks down a cookie or a piece of cake in exactly the same way that it does any other food. She explained that the food itself doesn't really matter. Instead, you just need to be in a 500 calorie deficit (see chapter 7) while eating the proper amount of nutrients to support optimal health if you want to lose weight or maintain your current weight.

I was still under the impression that if I wanted to see gains I would need to eliminate foods. I thought if I ate dairy or processed foods that I would start to gain weight. I was still seeing food as very black and white, good versus bad. (Side note, sometimes there can be truth to these statements. Dairy is notoriously hard on the gut, and processed foods as your main source of intake have proven not optimal fuel for your body in mass amounts over time.) The foundational truth was that my body wasn't keeping that score for me on the scale. I could still have bread and cheese, and as long as I was 500 calorie deficit I would lose weight.

This woman was making videos of herself cooking food while she took care of her twin toddlers. The difference was that she didn't look like any fitness and nutrition coach—she was absolutely ripped. Her muscles were defined and she looked strong and fit. She had incredible abs, and yet in her videos, she said that she still ate cookies. I was watching her thinking *I don't believe her*. I thought, *there is no way this woman is not hungry and has abs like that.* Honestly, the only people that I saw that looked like her—with defined muscles and a ripped physique—were bikini competition competitors. I knew the hard work it took for them to get that type of physique. They were not eating cookies. As a matter of fact, I was friends with some bikini competition competitors and I knew how restrictive their diets were. It wasn't freedom, and that is what I attached to my own ideas of what it takes to be lean. Maybe, just maybe, this woman was onto something I didn't see yet. I knew that I had to find out.

I was so curious that I wanted to sign up for one of her coaching programs. I wanted to learn more because I felt like she had valuable information. I was inspired by what she was teaching and since I was just finishing up nutritional therapy, I wanted to learn how other people were running their programs. I knew that I had a lot to learn from her.

I signed up and worked with one of her coaches for 12 weeks. I was eager to hear about how they taught people to have freedom from food. Throughout the twelve weeks, I mostly learned how to see food as neutral, not emotionally charged. I began to understand the beliefs that I had around things like *"this food is good"* and *"this food is bad"* or *"don't do this exercise"* and *"don't eat this food."*

The coach taught me to stop following plans that other people had set out for me, like training plans or nutrition plans that didn't include things that I really liked to do/eat. But rather, that I could create my own plan that would fit into my life for extended periods of time. A plan that was sustainable enough for me to be healthy and fit for years, not just for an upcoming event. Their coaching really showed me how to stop yo-yo dieting and stop thinking of my diet in terms of when I was "on the wagon" or "off the wagon." They helped me develop a plan and a viewpoint that meant that I was living my life to the fullest. This plan is what I do to show up and take care of myself every single day, not something that I start and stop. It was truly putting the power of consistency into everything that I did. Over time, it is consistency that breeds results. It is never about how perfect you could be until you fail and give up. How could I figure out a way to eat and move in a manner that I loved? That would be what allowed me to keep going no matter what.

Throughout the 12 weeks, I learned that there are no good or bad foods, just the quantities in which you consume the foods you like to eat. Some of your food is to fuel and nourish your body other foods are celebratory or for enjoyment and that's okay, too. It was more about understanding the process in which I could enjoy celebratory things within parameters that still allowed me to feel like I was meeting my goals.

They helped me develop a set of specific goals that weren't restrictive. Other diets I had done had been so restrictive. I would feel like I was "on the wagon" for 16 weeks, restricting all the foods that I loved and that tasted good to me. But when I did those types of diets, I found that when 16 weeks was over, I went just as hard eating all the things I had restricted from my diet. This was so different. They taught me ways to reach my goals by learning things I'd never learned before. Things like how to order at restaurants, and how to be social and healthy at the same time. I learned to ask myself questions like *do I have to drink all the time, or do I just drink because of social connection?* I learned how to travel and still keep my goals by being more intentional about what I wanted from the trip and how I wanted to feel coming home.

What I learned most in the program was how to play by my own rules and take a slow approach to moving the needle forward in the direction that I want. I learned that it's not realistic to say that I'll never have a cookie ever again. Furthermore, I learned that that kind of restriction backfired for me and turned food into an obsession. It's better to be real with yourself about when and why you want to enjoy the cookie.

I fell in love with the community of women in the coaching program. They took a different approach to fitness and nutrition. The participants and coaches all seemed to embody progress over perfection. This was an area where I really needed support. I loved that they were so focused on mindset. Up until this point, I do not think I had ever focused on the mindset I had as being important in personal results and success. However, when I started to reach my goals, I understood how differently I was approaching my thinking. It all starts with how you think. Our thoughts are energy, and over time, they show up in our physical world. Where you are today is in direct correlation to how you feel about yourself and what you think you deserve.

This coaching program helped me gain an understanding of the connection between our thoughts and our actions when it comes to nutrition and movement. Every other diet or nutrition plan that I'd tried only gave me instructions on what to eat and did not help me come up with a better mindset about food overall. Much of what I learned during those 12 weeks are the very same tools that I use today when working with my clients.

In this community, I learned to identify why I held certain beliefs around food and break those beliefs down. I learned from other people's stories and was able to discover some of my own beliefs that held me back. You need a community to rally around you. They help you push past times when you feel like you've come as far as you can on your own. When you feel safe with a group of people you trust, it pulls you towards a greater version of yourself. That's what I wanted. I wanted to get to a place that I had never been.

When it comes to change, it's important to understand the impact that social conditioning has on you. There are ways in which community can empower you to change, but also ways in which community can hold you back. When I was in the second grade, I was diagnosed with ADHD. I was put on Ritalin, which is dangerous if not taken properly. I had to do blood work and go to extra doctors appointments to make sure that the medication was working properly and that I was managing it well.

I remember that while in school, every time I was loud or even talked out of turn in the slightest way, my teacher would ask, "Have you taken your medicine yet?" So I'd take my medicine and very quickly start to feel really drugged up; sluggish, tired and off. What I heard my teacher saying to me was, "I need you to fit in in order to be in this classroom with us." It was another way in which I felt my differences made me unworthy. I was so hard on myself, always wondering why I couldn't just be like everyone else. This is a dangerous mentality for us to get stuck in. What actually *is* normal? And who defines it? As long as you believe normal exists outside of you, you will never value your own uniqueness.

Well, when I became an adult, I learned that I was misdiagnosed. I do not have ADHD at all. I'm just really smart and I was fucking bored in a classroom that wouldn't allow for me to share my thoughts or play or get anxious energy out through movement, something we all need to do at times. No, instead we are asked to suppress our true selves by the name of "normal." Instead of teachers trying to learn ways to challenge me, they just dug deeper into the social construct that all students must sit quietly to learn. This social construct hindered me in becoming who I wanted to be. My community was not only holding me back from being my true self, but I was also learning to take on their beliefs too, like *"a good student doesn't speak up."* I was silencing myself. This would become a pattern of survival for me for many years. Here's the thing, I hold no judgement for myself. Sometimes we *have* to survive. I did that and I did it well. But when surviving starts to impact our lives in a negative way, we must take a look and ask ourselves *does this way of existing serve me anymore?* If not, then it's time to ask, *what do I actually want now?*

Our environments are crucial. I've already mentioned that the top five people you spend your time with are the most likely to have the biggest influence on you. This could be a good or bad influence. If the people you spend your time with feed your negative thought loops or encourage you to give up on your goals, then you will likely do that. If the people you spend your time with are focused on balanced nutrition and strong mental/physical health, then you're likely to take those things seriously as well. It's human nature to do what your community is doing.

A study published in the *Journal of Consulting and Clinical Psychology* found that individuals who participated in a weight loss program that included an accountability group lost more weight and were more likely to maintain their weight loss over time compared to those who did not have the support of an accountability group. Similarly, a review of research on the effectiveness of accountability groups for improving health behaviors found that individuals who participated in an accountability group were more likely to adhere to their treatment regimens and make positive lifestyle changes compared to those who did not have the support of an accountability group.[i]

It's common for us to understand the need for accountability and community in some structures. If someone is addicted to drugs or alcohol, for example, and they desire change, they are going to need to find a supportive community of people. If your entire community is still using drugs or alcohol, it's going to be very hard to change. However, if a person who is addicted finds a different community—a support group of sober people or a sponsor who is sober—they can make progress toward their goals. They aren't alone. They are surrounded by people who have been in the same spot they have been and who have healed from their struggles. They can learn valuable lessons from a community of people who are sober as opposed to a community of people who are still using. In addition, there's a framework for them, a program to follow.

It's said that successful sobriety comes from following the plan, but also from staying in contact with that community. That means totally changing your life. It means changing where you go, how you do things and how you think about things. You have to become somebody completely different, but the benefits are huge and the gains far outweigh the losses. For someone with an addiction, getting sober means getting their life back, regaining bonds and relationships with family members, repairing issues at work, feeling more confident and stable, making healthy decisions, improving mental health—the list goes on.

The same happens when becoming a healthy, fitness-minded person who takes care of themselves. If you're in an environment where it's normal to forsake your health and repeatedly engage in unhealthy habits, it's going to be really hard to change your life. If you decide that being healthy is what you want to be and your environment doesn't support that, you might want to borrow belief. This might mean finding somebody specific—someone who has either done what you are aiming to do or who knows the ways to do it—who can provide the tools to navigate the situation. You can begin to develop the belief by simply leaning on someone else until you have zero emotional charge to engage in risky behaviors that don't support your overall goals.

When I found other women who saw the bigger picture of wanting to change their whole lives by being more active, energetic and happy, I was inspired. They gave me the belief that it was okay to accept myself as I am and understand that my differences are actually gifts. Before, I always felt like there was something wrong with me. I had altered my authentic self over and over again to try to fit into the social norms and expectations. This was true of my early motherhood experience, when I felt the obligations and the abandonment of my own self were crushing. I couldn't meet the expectations, but instead of trusting myself to find my own way, I just felt like a failure.

Once I found my community, there was a huge transition for me. I realized that it was better for me to be exactly who I am than to spend my whole life being somebody I'm not. When I was placating everyone else's needs and trying to fit into social constructs, I wasn't truly living. In fact, I was suffering. I like to say that I would rather love and bleed than not show up at all.

My weekly calls, online meet ups and check-ins made the biggest difference for me. This is the exact same method that I use when I'm coaching women, and it works. Over and over, I meet clients who have been at this thing alone. They've been trying to lose weight, change their habits around food or get energy back. Maybe they even just want to feel happiness again, and they've been alone through the process. It's exhausting for them to keep going, especially if they are doing something that hasn't helped them work through their mental blocks. They feel so isolated from the people around them. It's lonely. But once they find a coach or other support groups, they start to see some hope again. They realize that they don't have to do it alone, that there are tons of women out there who want the same things, who truly understand their struggles and who can help support them when they feel like giving up. Working with a group changes everything.

A mom came to me for coaching. She had two small children and felt overwhelmed with how much running around she was doing with her kids' schedules. At the end of the day, she had little time left for herself. She was struggling to lose fifteen pounds after being on a weight loss journey that had reached a plateau. She described feeling that she had lost touch with herself and she wasn't sure how to keep going on her own. She didn't know what to focus on or how to get motivated to keep going. She couldn't do this journey alone anymore; she needed community.

I help all of my clients work on their mindset while learning how to integrate health and nutrition into their lives as a foundation, not just something you do to get weight off quickly. It's hard for many of them, because they just want to lose weight or start feeling better right away. Our culture is so used to fad diets that doing anything that takes time sounds wrong. They want change so badly. It takes them time to come to terms with the "go slow to go fast" idea.

When learning new ideas or behaviors, my clients sometimes feel pressure that they have to do it perfectly or it will all come crumbling down. This is likely from years of conditioning that diets have to be restrictive to work. Many women think this because the word "diet" has come to mean so many negative things like hunger, deprivation and giving up foods that bring joy. When dieting, we've somehow mistaken the word for consistency with perfection and when we get off track, we feel we've failed. This leads us to the worst possible outcome giving up. When things don't go perfectly, we think things like *I tried and it didn't work* or *I can't work that hard with everything I've got going on in my life*. Perfectionism is not striving for excellence. It's not a superpower. Perfectionism is striving to meet an impossible standard that does not exist. It's completely unachievable. And according to *Psychology Today,* perfectionism increases the risk of health issues including eating disorders, anxiety disorders, pathological worry and premature death[ii].

We forget that life is not perfect. There are never going to be consistently smooth weeks or even days where nothing goes wrong. There's just so much outside of our control. Things come up, we forget our lunch at home, our kid gets sick, we get sick, we have to work late, we forget to get groceries, we get a flat tire.

It's dinner time and we're starving, so we finish off the kids' french fries instead of getting our macros for that meal; we feel like having cake and then we do. Perfection doesn't exist. That's why so many women tend to give up when they just can't do it perfectly.

I'll never forget this mom I was working with who was feeling nervous about her upcoming 40th birthday party in Las Vegas. We'd been working together for about 16 weeks and she had not yet worked on ways to be social and still remain fit in this new identity that she was cultivating. She didn't know how to go on vacation and still be healthy. Honestly, who really does in our society? Vacation traditionally means all fun and no boundaries!

I helped her dig a little deeper. We got to the bottom of her fear about messing up. She was scared to live life and have enjoyable moments because she didn't want to backtrack. She didn't know how to not do this new lifestyle of hers perfectly. I helped her understand her perfectionist mentality and revealed that perfectionism is a really low standard for ourselves. Life is not perfect. We are not perfect. We fluctuate daily, and so do our bodies, moods and behaviors. That's the reality. I held the mirror up for her so that she could see how this mindset was really holding back her progress.

I told her that I was glad she got to go to Vegas to celebrate her 40th birthday. I explained that if she messed up, that would be good! We need to learn how to keep going, how to keep showing up for ourselves, how to not be so depleted and in despair when we fluctuate on the scale from water weight or inflammation. We need to learn how to be consistent but also how to be in control of our choices when we want to celebrate. We need to know how to problem solve, lean into our struggles and build mental clarity and toughness. We cannot know this kind of resistance without things getting a little messy.

I explained to her that her birthday weekend was an opportunity to practice living the rest of her life. I taught her that failure is how we learn and how we can reflect and grow. It's how we know how to do things differently next time–that's what life is about. Is that easy? Heck no! If it was, everyone would be doing it. You can bet if something is worth doing, there will be growth and effort involved. When I work with clients in my community, I am more interested in what my clients have learned from their failures than how successful they've been or how perfect they were. Why does this matter to me so much? Because I've found that this is the biggest way we self-sabotage in general and stop before our goals and dreams are realized. We just get stuck in this loop that starts over and over. The best question you can ask yourself is *what if I just keep going?*

She explained to me that I helped take the pressure off of her shoulders. I helped her give herself grace, to honor her emotions and to trust herself. She let me know that she couldn't have done this alone. At the end of the year, she sent me a Christmas card that had a picture of her whole family smiling. She was taking photos again wearing the clothes that she felt good in. She felt connected to her two small kids and with her husband. She wrote in the card *"Thank you for helping me get my smile back!"* I still have that Christmas card today and I look at it to remind me why I do this work, why I keep showing up for this community and why it matters to keep showing up for myself. The resistance in our lives is a gut check for when it is time to change. If you are aware of what you resist, that's a good thing. It is time to change, not time to beat yourself up. It is time to dig in and do the work, the important work of growth and letting go of what no longer serves you.

In fitness, we do not have an information problem, but an application problem. If you're approaching a problem that you've never been successful with, it will be nearly impossible to resolve it without getting experienced help. Having accountability means everything to me and it means everything to my clients. I am definitely not saying that going at this alone will be impossible there are many people who have done that. I would just offer that for the majority of people, this is not the case. Everyone needs support and accountability of some kind. Going through this type of transformation can be isolating if other people in your life aren't on the same type of journey. People might judge you for meal planning constantly and always being prepared with your food on hand, or they might think that your non-negotiables about sleep and water are extreme. Having an accountability group of like-minded women working through the same goals really leveled up my environment. They were changing their mindset while I was changing mine.

We all have important intuition that we often suppress because of our social conditioning. For example, when I was working on becoming fit-minded, I had to go outside the box of what I was supposed to do. As a mom, there was just so much that needed to be done. I was conditioned to believe that I needed to keep a clean house, keep up with laundry, unload the dishwasher, attend all of my kids' activities, show up at school events and give my kids all of my time and attention. There was a lot of pressure to perform in the way that social constructs had laid out for me. But I wanted more than that. I wanted to work on things that a lot of moms weren't working on: my physical, emotional and spiritual health.

We ignore these desires or intuitions because they feel scary —or because we might not want to feel different. Sometimes what we're scared of is our own success. So we continue to suppress our true selves. But our inner desires will not die. When they are not honored, they come out in ways that are destructive. For example, it can play out in someone becoming an anxious mess, or someone turning to substances for relief from the suppression. This suppression can also turn into rage that is out of control and destroys healthy relationships. If you have no one around you that you can relate to or be real with, you might go back to your old habits and behaviors. The only thing that matters is our ability to be vulnerable with someone safe so that we can humble ourselves enough to be real and honest. For me, it was me allowing myself to tell the truth, to say *I am scared right now, I have never let myself get this far gone in my physical health, I need help*. We run from this type of vulnerability when we do not have a community safe enough to let our guard down.

When we desire change, we must have support. We need to see that someone else has done this and that they are safe. We need someone rooting us on and telling us that it's okay to keep going, to allow our true selves to emerge. At the very least, we need to find a group of people who understand why we might choose something different than the path everyone else is on. We need someone to say *"you are brave and you deserve this, so keep going."* To be loved in this way changes lives. I have watched it happen with so many women.

We are always creating. What you create and how well you perform starts in the patterns of your thoughts. If you're holding onto standards that are set by your community or a social construct that you no longer believe in, finding a community that aligns with your new belief system is going to matter. We must make a conscious effort to be in charge of our thoughts. We have to learn how to close negative loops and move forward with what we want now. This might mean that we need to learn how to become present and slow down enough to notice the belief systems of our environment and whether or not they are serving you. You will need to be mindful enough to see what you are creating or continuing within your thoughts. The more you are aware, the more authority you will have over the part you play in your creations, decisions and the influence you have over yourself.

For example, some belief systems that were likely built by social norms are:

- Something has to be hard in order to be able to gain progress.
- Some foods are bad and other foods are good.

- If it's easy, I'm not doing it right.
- I need food / alcohol to have fun.

When you find the right kind of coach and community, they can hold a mirror up to you and help you discover why you hold some of these untrue beliefs. I often ask clients why they think a cookie is bad and a salad is good. In actuality, a cookie has more nutrients than a salad. But salads have fewer calories than cookies, so you can eat more salad than you can cookies. That doesn't mean the cookie is *bad*—maybe you just have fewer to fit your goals for that day in order to see the success that you want. To cut a cookie out of your life because it is *bad* will only leave you feeling really restricted—and you will probably binge cookies when your willpower is broken. It is important to understand that building what you want (with parameters) is better for you in the long run. Salad fuels my body better because I can have more of it and I feel better after, but cookies are celebratory dense foods that I can still have. I may just need some parameters around how much and how often I eat cookies. Success is having something that works to meet my goals and lets me feel like I can have foods I love. I help clients learn how to see food as neutral so that they can begin to detach from the emotional charge that food brings up for them. In my community, the group will support this. They, too, are unlearning all the ways they have been wrongly taught to look at food and exercise. We unlearn to relearn, which results in positive actions and change. We learn what actually matters in the first place with nutrition as opposed to extreme diet culture. We actually take ownership of our own lives instead of following some mass produced plan that we don't even understand.

A community can count on each other and see themselves in each other's struggles. You can't change what you're not aware of. Sometimes others were able to point out things to me that I would have never seen on my own. Blocks, blindspots and negative thought loops are all normal challenges that would have been impossible to overcome alone.

If I ate out and didn't get to the gym, I might have felt like quitting, but accountability to others working toward the same goals kept me going. They helped me figure out what was really going on, helping me ask: Where was I blocked and what did I need? In addition, having a coach meant that I was getting tailored feedback on my exact progress and plan. All of it helped bring what was going on to the surface and helped me keep going, one vulnerable day at a time.

The community that I work with is designed for women to have professional support, help them dive deeper into mindset and habits and to encourage them to lean into the accountability aspect of life-changing behaviors. Having a group and community support also helps eliminate the chaos in your life. It helps build a strong foundation. That strong foundation will lead to building skills. It's about becoming consistent and dialing in the habits that will help you create a whole new identity. Over time, it's the community that helps challenge the status quo and encourages you to keep going when other people are doing things differently.

The community challenges you to find motivation and to participate when you feel overwhelmed. The community helps you determine obstacles and make plans. We learn from each other. When you see other people facing the same challenges, you can more easily answer questions like: *Who are the players in my life that can help me with this? What is the most crucial part of me to focus on? Where am I wasting my energy? How do I respond when I experience pressure?* You can learn from what they are learning. You can take hints, clues and other tips from those who have gone through this already. It helps us determine our blind spots.

Community is a powerful tool to help open up your eyes to different ways of looking at things. The other women are also there to step in when your mind won't stop telling you bad things about yourself. They will speak up when things are untrue, even when you've believed the lie you're telling yourself for a really long time. My clients tell me that the one thing I offer them when they have nothing left to give is that emotional support. They say that having someone who can push them when they need a boost or to sit with them while they work out their own blocks is what helps them make the transformation. They learn to have fun again and how to enjoy life while being healthy. For many women, this is just what they need: less seriousness and perfection, more real life. They learn that the journey they're on isn't about fitness, but becoming the best version of yourself. Community is vital to this growth.

There are many ways to find communities of support. Social media is a great way to find a community of people who are interested in the things that you are interested in. It's a great place to get started and it's usually free to follow alongside a professional who can give tips and tricks. There are also private, membership-based groups online that can be a great source of community. A gym is a great place to find community. People bond after doing a sweaty, fun workout. It's a great place to make friends in real life. You can start your own community, too. Gather together a group of women who want to work on the same goals as you do. Hold each other accountable via monthly coffee meetups or a text thread. Share your progress and root each other on. Take pictures of your balanced plates and send them to each other for recipe inspiration. Commit to holding up the mirror to each other, supporting each other in hard times and offering kindness when someone cannot offer it to themselves.

Takeaways

- Finding a community of people working on the same goals as you is vital to success.
- Community can help you see ways in which old thinking patterns are no longer useful.

- Community and accountability keep you motivated when you don't believe in yourself.
- Community can help show you ways that you might be self sabotaging when you can't see it for yourself.
- Community can help ensure that perfectionism is not holding you back.
- Community makes things more fun.

10 FINDING A LIFE WHERE YOU ARE FREE TO BE... JUST BE

FREEDOM IS ABOUT REACHING A PLACE IN YOUR LIFE WHERE YOU'VE been able to minimize as much resistance as possible. This comes with doing the work to automate habits you no longer have to think about—ie., they're no longer something you "have to do" and are now just "who you are." When you develop healthy habits that you do without any planning or thinking, you now have the bandwidth for more personal growth and development.

Freedom is an active process, one you will have to engage in as long as you walk the earth. It is a process of knowing your boundaries with others and yourself, and setting the parameters that guide and shape your world. It is a process in which you create an active state of feeling free. It's taken me a long time to realize that the resistance we experience in our lives is also a guide shaping us. We may feel "in flow" or free in one season and not in another. This means maybe something changed or shifted in our physical, mental, emotional or spiritual world that needs to be addressed. In other words, freedom isn't something that once sustained, is never thought of again. There is an ebb and flow to it, much like the changing of seasons. I truly feel like accepting this is part of the process of finding who you are and who you still want to be. Freedom isn't a place that once you've arrived, you never have to travel to again. It is a conscious daily effort to take care of yourself. You do this by staying curious about the things that you need in order to evolve and protect what you have created in your life that matters so much to you. This is a very active place to be.

I've talked about mindset a lot throughout this book. Your thoughts truly are what you will become. What you believe to be true about yourself is what you think about most. These beliefs subconsciously "drive the bus," and you manifest them in your physical world. Change happens when you address what you believe to be true of yourself and what you are capable of. As we come to the end of this book, I want to reiterate all the ways in which our negative thoughts keep us from living a life of freedom. One of the best books that I've read, and one that really encapsulates the power of mindset, is *The Mountain Is You* by Brianna Wiest. She writes about the concept that you are the mountain you are trying to overcome. In other words, *the obstacle is the way*. Instead of embracing the obstacles, we tend to approach life thinking that our obstacles are outside determining factors—someone or something else's fault. Often, we believe the thoughts and beliefs of other people and take those on as our own.

At the end of the day, everything you want is on the other side of the hard stuff that you are willing to walk through. It's not easy–it's brave. Let me tell you, anything worth doing will not be easy, otherwise everyone would be doing it. There are some things that will be the bravest things you've ever done; things like changing your life, your mindset, your circumstances and your finances. Changing your body is no different from the rest of the hard things we face. What you want to accomplish is on the other side of taking an honest look at and responsibility for where you are in this moment. In order to change, you have to set up some order in your life to make that effort. We can't focus on failures. We can't live in the past. Brianna Wiest says, "What if you knew that you were never meant to get it right the first time, but to build it through trial and error? How much more grace would you give yourself, how much more human might you be?....." I love those words and I like thinking about what I'm willing to do, knowing that it's the effort that counts. What if the goal isn't lost? What if everything up to this point has been the research you needed to change your life? It's the process of learning what you want, because you are so familiar with what no longer serves you.

In order to do this, we must first step outside of "the matrix," the illusion that our lives are already set in stone, that nothing can change. "The matrix" is the place where we still think that something has to be hard or that only *certain people* can go far in life. The truth is that you can go far in life. Your life is waiting for you to step out of "the matrix" into that reality, but no one can do it for you. Stepping outside of "the matrix" means completely unplugging from the beliefs that you've learned and adopted. You must decide that you want to discover your own set of beliefs. You must want to become self-aware. This is uncomfortable because it involves confronting truths about ourselves that we might not be ready to acknowledge. It means that we might have to own up to the fact that some of our problems are actually self-inflicted. It means that we must challenge our self-image. Sometimes this can be really difficult to do.

Many of these negative thoughts and beliefs are things that you took on as a child and have carried with you until now. Sometimes you don't even know it's happening. You don't realize that the negative thought loop running in the back of your mind is sabotaging everything you've ever wanted. There are countless examples, from fear of failure so you don't try, perfectionism so you don't finish or even not believing you are enough so you stop wanting anything more at all. You deserve to be happy, feel good and always choose more for yourself. You deserve a life where you follow through until you get what you want and need. We all do! These adopted beliefs are always trying to communicate with you. This is where you experience self-defeating thoughts like *maybe I'm not good enough for this.* What we truly believe deep down is the place from which we develop vices that help us cope. These can be things like pushing people away, dwelling in the past, caring more about what others think, spending too much money, mindlessly scrolling through social media or using emotional eating to numb these thoughts. In order for change to occur, you have to be present enough to take a good hard look and see that you are worthy, loved and safe. Maybe there's trauma or overwhelm that needs to be addressed so that you can learn some more healthy coping skills and don't self-sabotage when things become hard.

For any kind of change to happen, we have to be aware of our negative thought loops, address them and reshape them and the negative actions that follow. For example, develop an understanding of why you might have self defeating thoughts. It could be a defense mechanism, a belief that if you think badly about yourself first, then you won't be blindsided by someone else thinking badly about you. You punish yourself for having big dreams, ambitions and goals by saying to yourself *I could never do that.* Then you engage in actions that reinforce your thoughts, actually doing the opposite of your goal.

Another example of a negative thought loop that could be sabotaging your success is pushing people away. Instead of joining a support group or finding a community, you choose to do things alone. This is a form of isolation. It can be from trauma, like hurt from a past rejection. You protect yourself from a person or a group that can help you because you're afraid of getting hurt again. You're too afraid to be vulnerable enough to be your true authentic self. It's such a detriment to progress, because it's only once you fully love and accept yourself that others can love you for who you really are. We cannot know this until we lean in and learn to process our emotions in a different way than before. That is what true change and true healing means.

Another negative thought loop is feeling overwhelmed.

Sometimes as women, we put everyone and everything in front of ourselves. We care for our children, for our neighbors, for our communities, our partners, our parents, and at the end of the day we have nothing left to give. This leads to exhaustion, impulsivity and apathy when it comes to nutrition and movement. Maybe that means eating poorly when we intended to eat macronutrients, or not drinking enough water throughout the day. Maybe we stay up extra late to get some time to ourselves, but that backfires, because it means we're too tired to get up in the morning and work out before having to care for everyone again. This leads to mental overload. You lack nourishment, rest and movement which are all essential for your brain to get the right chemicals to make you feel stable and happy. If you give all you have to everyone else, then who is taking care of you? Who is making sure that you are living the life you desire? This can lead to emotional hunger. You lack the life-giving experiences you crave. You have basic emotional needs; we all do. We cannot decide to show up and need less. It will always come out in some contorted way. We must do the work of identifying what we need and learn to be vulnerable enough to get those needs met.

Another major factor that inhibits people from going big with their goals and dreams is fear. You might automatically think and believe what you feel in terms of worry and doubt. For example, you worry that something will be hard, and therefore it *is* hard. Or you believe that something is going to be too scary, so then it *does* actually feel scary. You become what you believe, and fear is the biggest culprit hindering your progress. Maybe fear is more comfortable because that's what you're used to. Instead of trusting your intuition and relying on your gut, you blindly trust everything that passes through your mind. You trump your gut to the point that you disconnect from your true essence—and then you no longer trust what your gut is telling you. This, my friend, is a dangerous place to be. However, it happens to us all at one point or another.

It's important to remember that your brain lies to you. It's trying to keep you safe at all times, and it doesn't know the difference between the perception of fear and actual fear. When we're in a situation we perceive as threatening (such as changing our whole lives), our bodies respond by motivating us to react in one of three ways: run away as fast as possible (flight), fend off an attack (fight) or stay motionless to avoid detection (freeze).[i] In order to get past fear, you have to work with your mind to stop fearful thoughts from becoming reality. You have to realize that not every thought you have needs all of your attention. If you feel scared about trying a new workout, for example, you have to quiet those thoughts by using mindfulness practices or meditation. The more you practice quieting your fear, the better you will become at overcoming your fears and taking action.

Identifying self-sabotaging patterns begins with being more aware of what you don't want then what you do want. You need to ask yourself *What do I want in my life? How can I live a life where I'm thriving?* This is where we start to gain emotional intelligence: the ability to understand, interpret and respond to our emotions in a healthy way. Your brain was designed quite literally to keep you safe, and if you don't work with your mindset, you might find that what you resist, persists. I encourage clients to take a deeper dive into their thoughts, behaviors and actions to make sure they take the steps they need to build the lifestyle they desire.

Stepping outside of "the matrix" comes with constant evaluation of what it is that you're experiencing and asking yourself *Is this belief my own? Where is it coming from? If it's not my own, why is it still here? Is this belief trying to keep me safe or comfortable? Is it okay for me to explore a new idea and try different behaviors?*

You may have heard the phrase "heal your inner child" in regards to mental health and healing practices. In an article from *Cleveland Clinic*, psychologist Susan Albers explains that healing your inner child is about learning how to move forward. When you heal your inner child, you rediscover what you need, recapture what you've lost and reparent your younger self so you can heal from past experiences.[ii] This usually looks like reconnecting with a past event/time in which you were hurt as a child and then giving that child (you) what you needed back then. Sometimes it's the reassurance that everything is going to be okay, safety, a hug, a smile or something deeper, depending on your personal experience.

Growing up, I spent a lot of time not being very kind to myself. I spent a lot of time in fear. I rarely let the adults in my life in on what was happening inside my mind, and so sometimes that meant that my needs went unmet. Or even worse, I tried suppressing my needs thinking that I could have less needs as a means to survive. Some of the things that happened to me felt traumatic, and because I never asked for help, I began to develop some limiting self beliefs. These were things like: *you just can't get it right, there's something wrong with you, you're the only one like this, you are too much for people and if you tell them you're struggling, you will ultimately be abandoned.*

Instead of working through these beliefs, I carried them with me right into adulthood. Every time I was faced with a difficult situation, a relationship that was complicated, my body issues, I would have these same thoughts: *there is something wrong with me* or *I'm not like everyone else.* These feelings affected the way I felt about myself. They reflected back to me that I was all wrong. These beliefs affected how I coped, how I lived and how I used food especially. I was stuck.

It wasn't that long ago that I would walk by a mirror, unable to look at the person staring back at me. I was depressed, filled with anxiety and had no zest for life. I was in a dark place. My negative loops running in the background and constantly sabotaging me were all about my self worth. Somewhere deep down, I didn't think that I deserved to feel better. So anytime I would start to make progress, I would find a way to sabotage it by either giving up, binging or engaging with people who reflected back to me how I felt myself. For things to change this time around, I couldn't just go on another diet. That wasn't the solution. I had to go much deeper than that. I had to work through my entire belief system. I had to look back over my entire life to find out how I developed these beliefs about myself; from the time my mom said something about my size, to my attempts and failures at perfection, to my self isolation as a tool for no one ever having to see the real me. I had never reached so deep before to try and change the narrative.

Over the years, I've done deeply healing work. I've learned to sit with hard emotions that I used to shove down or pacify. I've developed an understanding of where those beliefs came from and began to see that they were not mine and that they were not helping me anymore. Because of the work I've done, I've had some major breakthroughs. Recently, I went back to my childhood home. Usually when visiting I don't sleep in my childhood bedroom alone. Either we rent a place nearby or I have a kid or two sleeping in there with me. This time I was alone in the bedroom I grew up in as a child. That night, while everyone else was asleep, I was lying in bed journaling. Right before bed, I turned off the light and in the silence of the dark room, I heard my inner child. I heard what sounded like Emily's little voice. She said, "You came back for me."

I bolted up out of bed and stood in the room looking around. I was moved by the voice that I heard. Through the darkness, my eyes landed at a spot in the room where I remember crying dramatically as a child. I looked straight at that spot and I said,

"I came back for you Em."

It was the most profound and powerful experience I've ever had. In that moment, I realized that I saved myself. I thought, *I'm a fucking warrior*! It was like something inside of me shifted, and I knew that I didn't have to go back to being the little girl who felt all wrong anymore. Now, I can trust myself to move forward and take care of myself.

Throughout this process, I have learned that emotionally healthy people have a flexibility to their psyche. That is something that can be developed in anyone. It starts with awareness, asking questions and slowly building the resilience that leads to adaptability, problem-solving and self-soothing. We must expect failure and use it as a tool to help us get closer to what we desire. We have to plan, execute and evaluate constantly. And when we do, miracles happen.

Freedom for me means that I've followed through with my commitment to myself. For nutrition, it means that I've decided how I want to eat and what I like to eat that will leave me feeling like my best self. If I choose to celebrate and enjoy foods or drinks that don't leave me feeling my most optimal, that's okay. I'm not starting anything over or quitting anything. When I'm finished celebrating with food or drink, the next moment, I'm right back to doing the things that matter to me, eating foods that fuel and support my body. I am making sure that I get enough sleep. I'm making sure that I'm eating enough protein, fruits and vegetables. I'm minimizing processed foods. I am hydrating.

Freedom in movement means that I never wonder how or when I'm going to "get my workout in." Instead, movement is something that I do everyday and is part of my daily practice. I have now moved so often and so frequently that not moving would be harder than getting up to exercise. This doesn't mean it has to be perfect. If I don't feel like lifting weights one day, I'll ask myself, *what do I feel like doing?* and then follow through with what feels good to me in that moment.

Freedom in my mind is having a toolbox of skills that I can turn to when my mind plays tricks on me. It's understanding how my thinking patterns create my reality. It's knowing who I can call and what kind of help I can ask for when I need it. It's knowing that I don't have to do this thing alone anymore–I've got support.

When I told my friend that I was going to change my whole fucking life after leaving my doctor's appointment that day, I didn't know how or where I would start. All I had to do was begin, do one thing that moved me closer to what I wanted. Eat one meal with vitamins and minerals, go on one 10-minute walk, rest instead of folding laundry, and when negative self thoughts came up for me, reframe them. I had to do the hardest thing–commit to myself and go slow. I had to start small and celebrate each little victory. I just kept focusing on the next day, and then the next day, to get to a place where I finally felt was good enough. This built momentum. My new thought was: *Maybe I can just keep going.* Then I lost 25 pounds, 30 pounds, 50 pounds —all the way up to losing 80 pounds. When I looked at myself, I realized that it wasn't just looking good that made me happy. Really, I was just so damn proud of myself! I was responsible for turning my life around and my whole family's life around, and it made me feel incredible.

We're not trying to be carbon copies of each other. We're trying to do things that make us come alive and feel alive. I'm free now because I have learned how to set up my life in a way that promotes health and growth in every season of life. On our team, we talk about what to focus on when we're feeling our best but more importantly, what to focus on during difficult times. We encourage clients to ask themselves *what are two to three things you know you need to do to take care of yourself that are not negotiable?* Freedom is knowing that on your hardest days, you will not fail your physical, mental or spiritual health. Maybe the three things are as simple as sleep, hydrate and walk. These little things will help you feel better on hard days and ensure that you are still making progress. When you feel better, you do better and you will begin to gain momentum that will change your life forever. If you just keep going, eventually you will be able to work effortlessly towards the life that you want.

Everyone on Earth is on a diet: if you eat food, then you have a diet. When I was young, my diet consisted of processed foods and whatever casserole my mom would serve to me. As I grew a little older, my diet became restrictive and damaging. Today, I'm still on a diet—but this time, it's made up of the right kind of foods, foods that my body needs to function optimally.

I'm not here to just exist; I'm here to live my life to the fullest —and thanks to everything I've been through and all that I've learned, I have so much freedom. I'm free from yo-yo diets, free from binging and guilt, free from shame, free from self-hatred and low self-worth. Free from gaining and losing weight over and over again. Free from the fear that I will gain the weight back. My mind is free from negative loops and unhelpful narratives that keep me stuck. I am free to be whoever I want to be.

Today, I know how to take care of myself in ways that I never did before. I wake up in the morning before the rest of the house so I can take time to cultivate my mind and my soul. This sets up my emotions for the day. I have a coffee and I'll journal. I read something from my favorite book to continue to grow my mind. This way, I can connect with myself before I start taking care of anyone else for the day. This allows me to show up and be the mom I want to be and have the energy for my family.

This also helps build my resilience on the hard days. I think one of the greatest things that has happened in taking care of myself is that I've become a lot more flexible than I've ever been. My ability to self-soothe has grown. I now have a greater capacity to handle disappointment, to work through conflict with friends, to understand *hey I might not feel good today—but I have the knowledge and skills to be able to work through these challenges.*

This makes the good days and the "mountains" so much sweeter. I have developed an environment full of people who pour into me, who support me and who love me. I'm understanding what healthy relationships look like. I'm finding people who finally reflect back to me the beauty in me. I still focus on movement and exercise. I like strength training and do it often. I love doing Pilates and I love to play tennis. I've made wonderful friends doing these things that I love. I am still focused on eating lean meat, fruits and vegetables and food that fuels my body while building muscle at the same time. Nutrition and movement have given me my life back, and so I continue to focus on a healthy and fit mind and body.

I'm really living in the same way that I ask my clients to live. Although my vision boards look different, I'm still doing them. Now, my goal is to get one percent better than yesterday, one percent better than last week, one percent better than last year. I'm constantly asking myself *how can I continue to grow?* I once heard someone say that if you're not embarrassed by some of the things you did or said or by some of your choices from last year, then maybe you're not growing enough. That's my goal now: *just be better than Emily was before.*

All of this work has allowed me to live from this amazing authentic space and people are drawn to authenticity. It's the highest vibration that you can be. By living my authentic truth, I give people the freedom to think: *well, let me try to see who I am too.* I want everyone I work with to feel this way. I want to provide a safe enough space for people to open up and figure out who they are, because unless you feel safe, you will never be as vulnerable as you need to be to find out what is lurking under the surface.

I'm finally confident, not just in my body but in my mind. I exude confidence. When I'm feeling this confident, I give people permission to be who they are as well. I have this friend who is so uniquely herself that it's captivating. I told her once, *"Thank you for living your life in such a way that it makes the rest of us brave."* I think people are hard on one another because we're hard on ourselves. What if we let ourselves go in such a way that we radiate to others the ability and the draw to do the same? I think that's actually the beauty of being a woman. It's so far beyond how we look. Sure, looking beautiful is fine, but life is really about cultivating beautiful gardens in our souls that allow us to be feminine yet strong. Women are the best supporters of one another; when we're operating from a healthy space, we can thrive. This is what I try to help women with and what I want women to find in themselves. When you've walked through fire, you want to turn back around and hand buckets of water to the others still walking through it.

I would be doing other women a disservice if I didn't share my story. Women need to hear that it's possible for true change and growth to take place in all of our lives. They need to know that you're never too far gone to give yourself another chance at life. This isn't about weight loss. It's about learning the way that your individual body works. What foods make you feel good, what movements will give you the most endorphins, what coping skills will manage stress, what steps need to be taken to manage hormone health and more. There is no one-size-fits-all; it's all totally customizable and only you have the blueprint.

Sure, looking good felt fun, but that was the short-term gain. What I gained internally from this journey and the person I became—the resilience, the confidence, the improved relationships, the strong mental health—is what truly enhanced my life.

Ladies, the time to take care of yourself is now. There is no other time more necessary than the moment you are in. If that moment happened to pass you by and you didn't change anything, then choose the next moment. A recent article from the *New York Times* highlighted the burden of motherhood and how it affects women's health. The article described a tired mom, who at the end of a long day, carved out enough time to get some movement in. After constant interruption from her kids, however, she finally gave in and decided to help them with their needs over working out and meeting her own. The author writes: "It's a story that's played out in millions of homes, as women feel pulled between taking care of themselves and taking care of family. In a study of 400,000 Americans, only 33 percent of women met weekly recommendations for aerobic exercise, as opposed to 43 percent of men."[iii]

I can specifically remember when this was true for me. As women and mothers, we often have no space as we continue to shoulder the emotional and physical demands of the home. This could not have been more true for me. Before having children, I could work out whenever I wanted. I was free to do whatever I liked with my time, at my leisure. If I felt like sleeping in and working out at night, I could do that. If I felt like going to the gym at three in the afternoon, I could do that too. Now as a mom, the idea of having time to workout at night or during after school pickup time seems impossible. There is no way that I could do either of those things.

There was a time when both of my kids were babies and I remember my spouse going to the gym for two whole hours. No one noticed that he was gone. The major burdens of the household fell to me. I was breastfeeding. I was the default parent when the babies cried. I knew all the things that they needed and when they needed them. When we left for a trip, all my husband needed were his keys and his suitcase. I had to find the breast pump and all the parts, get the baby bag packed, make sure that the right size clothes were packed with the right stuffed animals and pacifiers. The burden fell to me so much that I would often choose to stay home. Looking back, I realized not only did the burden fall on me, I also let it. I didn't ask for help. I was trapped because I allowed myself to be.

When I went to the gym, I felt rushed to get back and guilty that I was taking up too much time. There were times that I would feel resentful. It is only now that I can see that resentment carried an intelligence with it. I had a need and it was not getting met. I have a responsibility to ask for what I need. Otherwise, I will resort to blaming someone else. When we had kids, he could effortlessly carry on with his life, mostly in the same way that he had before. For me, everything changed. Or at least in my mind. I was hyper-focused on the ways it changed. I couldn't see the value of what I had or how to move through it like I do now. All the ways in which I used to cope were gone. I felt this crushing pressure that I had to put my babies first and myself last.

The *NYT* article explains that putting yourself last in terms of exercise is not good for your health. "Over time, this exercise shortfall can have serious implications on women's health. While women live an average of six years longer than men, they spend a greater percentage of their lives in poor health, suffering from conditions like heart disease, diabetes or depression." Can you read that statistic again? We live longer, but we are on average suffering, and we do not have to! Ladies, it doesn't have to be this way.

Having PPD opened my eyes to this. It made me realize how severely my health could fade if I chose not to take care of myself. While PPD is not something that you can completely avoid with health and fitness, proper self care can greatly reduce the symptoms. I needed to prioritize myself first and reframe the idea that taking care of myself first is selfish. Taking care of oneself is actually the greatest form of love one can possibly demonstrate.

It's estimated that it costs families about $15k per year to raise a child. These include expenses for housing, food, education, healthcare and transportation. When I'm working with mothers, many of them seem to have no problems spending money for their children's healthcare needs like braces, checkups and sports physicals. When it comes to investing in themselves however, they consider it a luxury. Many women feel like spending money for exercise (to join a gym) or on nutrition (like a nutritional meal plan) is frivolous and can only be considered once everything else is paid for. Quite frankly, these are the women who don't really want to invest in themselves. According to the article, only four percent of mothers considered their own health as a measure of their success, while 31 percent saw their children's health in these terms.

I explained in chapter eight how important movement is to longevity. Having the physical ability to walk, carry your groceries in the house, go up stairs and pick up your grandchild will depend greatly on how well you take care of yourself now. If you're not building strength and mobility now, you may be at higher risk for injury and illness later. It will matter to your kids then too. If you cannot engage with your grandchildren by going to their sporting events or playing with them outside, your kids will notice. It's not a luxury to move your body, it's essential! Oftentimes, it seems like we have our whole life ahead of us but really there are no guarantees. Taking care of your longevity starts now. It's essential whether you think so or not. One day, your health will remind you of the ways in which you did or didn't take care of yourself.

The same goes for nutrition. It's essential to make time for nutrition in your life. Planning what you will eat and how you will get macronutrients isn't superfluous. It's vital to living the life of your dreams. There are essential nutrients that your body needs and does not make on its own so you have to eat them–vitamins A, B, D, C and K, to name a few. More and more studies are showing that what we eat now, in our forties and fifties, matters later in life. A Harvard study, based on data from over 100,000 people spanning 30 years, revealed that people who followed a healthy diet from their 40s onward were 43-84 percent more likely to be well-functioning physically and mentally at age 70 compared with those who did not.[iv] This is something to consider if you plan to put off your health until the kids are grown. It might be too late.

I can't say enough about how important nutrition and movement are for women, especially moms. There is so much evidence that taking care of the most basic essentials will go a long way in your overall health. There is also so much evidence showing women on average put themselves last. We are suffering, ladies. The greatest thing you can do for your families, and to impact your world for the better, is to take care of yourself. You first, then others. Just like safety regulations on the airplane, your oxygen mask goes on first; otherwise you cannot breathe in order to help someone else.

There's more, though, and it's not just about being healthy and looking thinner. When you focus on the foundations of your life, starting with the most basic things, everything else starts to improve. When you take care of yourself by moving and eating the proper nutrients, you will feel better. When you feel better, you will make better decisions, which might mean going for a walk with a friend instead of folding laundry. The walk will lead to endorphins that will lead to feelings of happiness. The connection with your friend will lead to feelings of fulfillment, joy and maybe even laughter. When you bring that joy back into your home, you have better interactions with your children. You quite literally create more positive energy in your life and for others by doing so. Let the mess slide for once and choose to connect instead. The ripple effect that these small (but crucial) actions and decisions have on your life can become so big that, before you know it, you've changed your life. You have become the best version of yourself. I know this because it happened to me. It sneaks up on you in the best of ways and you are able to see how the path of resistance, the work you are avoiding, is the path you must walk. The trails you must blaze through the overgrown field of life pave the way for change.

Once I took my health and wellness back into my own hands and took tiny steps forward every day, new opportunities opened for me at different intervals along my journey. With each opportunity, I had the choice to keep moving the needle forward just a bit or stay in the same place. I didn't have the option of going back my babies needed me. I will never regret doing the hard work that it took to get me here. Not every day is easy. There are times when my motivation is low or I don't feel my best, but I show up anyway. I know what it's like to give up. I already know the outcome of letting myself get too far away from my true authentic self: I start to let those negative thoughts creep back in, I become consumed with my body and I get distracted with quick fixes or over-promised and undelivered solutions. In other words, "the matrix" sucks me back in. Today, I keep going to see what new opportunities will open to me, to discover where else I can grow and to learn how to better myself and my community. I encourage you to choose your path, too. If this book called out to you at all, then maybe you know deep down that you are made for more. The best revelation I have found is that no one is coming for you, so it's up to you! How amazing is that? No one else can carve out a life that feels like yours but you. Go and get what's yours!

Takeaways

- In order to have freedom, you must understand your belief system.
- What work does your inner child need from you?
- Own your beliefs and explore where some of your long-held beliefs come from.
- Set up a framework for how you are going to operate in the world and stick with it.
- Know your non-negotiables.
- Keep growing, learning and exploring.
- There is no limit.
- The time to start taking care of yourself is now.

AFTERWORD

In our society, we are so caught up with looking good that in that desperate fight, we can forget the most basic need of taking care of our bodies. I am talking about all that is connected in our body—heart, mind and soul. This goes far beyond the shell of our physical appearance. Our bodies are supposed to look phenomenal because of the great care that we take of them. We should not be apologizing for that. It is so much more than fitting into a pair of jeans or a number on a scale.

Nutrition and fitness matter. Many of the problems that women face can be improved by eating the right kind and right amount of nutrients. Often, though, true nutrition and fitness gets confused with dieting—and people often mistake losing weight for being healthy. I know I did. I thought being thin was the ultimate goal. I had no idea the impact that our diet has both on our physical health and also our mental health. The years of poor nutrition and lack of education about women's health left me blindsided by severe postpartum depression and a weight gain that seemed incomprehensible.

After hitting rock bottom, I realized that there was no one coming to save me. I had to be the person to take the steps to heal. That started by working on my mindset, then on nutrition, then on learning to move again. Slowly over time, I began to lose not just the weight, but also the faulty belief systems that I'd held onto for years. I transformed my life.

The skills I learned along this journey are invaluable. My hope is to inspire women by reshaping their belief systems, building their confidence, helping them understand how food works in the body and helping them develop exercise and fitness routines that feel good on a personal level. My outcome has been so positive that I now lead hundreds of other women through life-changing methods to help them create lives full of vitality. Lives where they feel confident to take up space, wear clothes that make them feel good, be in the rooms that they want to be in and do what they love.

TESTIMONIALS

Testimonials from Emily's clients:

"Working with Emily has been an absolute blessing. I was introduced to her as my personal development coach at a time when I deeply needed support in my fitness and nutrition journey. But what I gained from our time together was so much more than that.

I met Emily during a tender season of life, and from the very beginning, she met me exactly where I was. We connected over our shared love for fitness, the challenges of postpartum, the mental load of motherhood, our faith, and our passion for helping others. She created a space where I felt seen, heard and supported.

Each week, Emily encouraged me, challenged my perspective and helped me reframe my struggles in a way that felt empowering. She taught me to take control of what I could, trust the process and ultimately trust myself. Her vulnerability and willingness to share her own experiences made her guidance even more impactful—her honest and relatable stories became lessons that helped me grow.

While my physical transformation was evident, my mental

transformation makes me the most proud. People who have known me for years comment on how my energy has changed, and I truly believe that Emily's guidance, along with the hard work and encouragement of the program and community, made all the difference.

Emily's unwavering support helped me find joy again. She is warm, funny and real. She leads with her heart and pours everything into those she works with. She isn't just an incredible coach—she is a true friend, and I'm endlessly grateful for the light she has helped me rediscover."

– Natalie R.

"I cannot recommend Emily enough! Working with her has been a life-changing experience. Emily took the time to understand my goals, challenges and personal preferences. Her guidance has been so practical and tailored to my specific needs. I've learned not only how to make healthier choices but also how to stay motivated, even on the tough days. Emily's support has been consistent and encouraging, and I always feel like I have someone in my corner. She has helped me reframe when needed, and look at food—and my relationship with food—in a completely different manner, providing tools that make this sustainable for the long game. The progress I've made, both physically and mentally, is beyond what I thought was possible. Emily has helped me build a sustainable lifestyle that works for me, and I'm feeling stronger, more confident and more energized than ever. She allows a safe space to really work through all of the challenges I faced mentally and physically. She is knowledgeable, supportive and straight up with me. If you're looking for someone who truly cares about your well-being and will work with you every step of the way, Emily is the person you need."

– Alaina O.

"Emily is, without a doubt, one of the most genuine people I have ever met. Though we've spent time together in person fewer than five times, the connection we share is among the strongest and most supportive friendships I have. Her results with clients speak volumes when it comes to physical transformation—but it's her emotional support that truly sets her apart from other coaches.

Emily shows up as her real, authentic self, and in doing so, she creates a space where you feel safe enough to be your real self, too. She has this incredible way of knowing exactly when to push you and when to let you sit with discomfort—long enough to experience those major breakthroughs you need. Whether you're riding the highs or navigating the lows, Emily is always there: listening, supporting and guiding.

One of my favorite things about Emily is that she always brings the fun. When we're together in person, we laugh until we cry. And when we can't be in the same room, she still finds ways to remind me that even though we're doing real work, we don't have to take ourselves too seriously. She has this gift for mixing joy with growth, making the journey both meaningful and enjoyable.

What makes Emily exceptional is that she doesn't just talk the talk—she walks the walk. She's constantly working on herself, attending masterminds, exploring new areas of growth and then bringing back everything she learns to benefit her clients. Watching her transform not only her own life but also the lives of others has been truly inspiring.

Working with Emily isn't just about fitness; it's about becoming the best version of yourself—and having a lot of fun along the way. For that, I'll always be grateful."

– Kate L.

"When I started working with Emily, I was 15 pounds heavier than I had ever been and I was on four different types of medication. I felt terrible all of the time. I had tried a ton of fad diets

and workouts and nothing would ever stick. At our first meeting, I remember wincing when I told Emily I just wanted to get back to my original weight and lose the 15 pounds...like it was a job too big to overcome. She did not hesitate and said that would be easy. After six months, I had lost 17 pounds. I've managed to get off 3 of the 4 medications, and my dose on the last medication has been cut in half. I've learned so much from her—not just about food and exercise, but about attitude and how important it is to not be scared or overwhelmed with the thought of either of them. She literally changed my life and I'm forever grateful!"

– Taylor S.

ACKNOWLEDGMENTS

I would like to thank my family for the support that they have shown me over the years, and the freedom to always chase my dreams even when the path wasn't always easy or clear. To my mom, who is always willing to work out every single issue we ever face together, and grow stronger in love. I would like to thank my kids for being the initial reason—then and now—for reminding me what unconditional love is, and how I have to have it for myself first. I would like to thank Jamie Gilley for brainstorming and vision planning with me every January about who and what we can be with no judgment and no competition, just love and friendship. I would like to thank Angie and Paul Lyngso for sharpening these concepts in me, and allowing me to have a platform to share my story and pulling from the amazing framework they have built together with nutrition and fitness, through years of blood, sweat and tears.

I would like to thank Anna David and all her amazing and talented team at Legacy Launch Pad for treating me with love and acceptance as I relived some hard moments in my life, and made it okay to be vulnerable and gave me permission to share my story with whoever needs to hear it. Namely, to Samantha Perkins, for working with me countless hours to capture my voice and put it in an amazing format of love.

To all the amazing coaches and mentors I have worked with from fitness, nutrition and leadership development: thank you for all you have given me and the safe space to evolve, grow, and most importantly, heal.

Last but not least, thank you to all the clients and women I have had the honor and privilege of working with. Thank you for inspiring me every single day with your resiliency to show up for your own lives through countless obstacles we all face as women. Thank you for living your lives in such a way that it makes the rest of us brave! I am forever changed by being your coach.

CITATIONS

1. THE DARKNESS WAS ALL TOO CONSUMING

i. Mayo Clinic, "Postpartum Depression - Symptoms and Causes."

2. HOW IT ALL BEGAN: GROWING UP IN THE '90S

i. Lee, "Why the USDA Food Pyramid diet recommendations changed."

ii. UAB Medicine, "MyPlate Healthy Eating Chart Replaced the Food Pyramid."

iii. Reales-Moreno et al. "Ultra-Processed Food and Drinks Consumption Is Associated with Psychosocial Functioning in Adolescents."

Mesas et al. "Increased Consumption of Ultra-Processed Food Is Associated with Poor Mental Health in a Nationally Representative Sample of Adolescent Students in Brazil."

Samuthpongtorn et al. "Consumption of Ultraprocessed Food and Risk of Depression."

4. I MISS FOOD

i. Lebow, "Emotional Drinking: Are You Using Alcohol to Feel Better?"

ii. BrainsWay, "Why Do I Overeat When I Feel Depressed?"

6. IF NOTHING CHANGES, NOTHING CHANGES

i. Garza, "Postpartum Depression and Its Long-Term Effects on Children."

ii. EveryStep, "Postpartum Depression is Driving Maternal Mortality."

iii. CDC, "CDC Activities: Improving Maternal Mental Health Care."

iv. Leahy, *The Worry Cure: Seven Steps to Stop Worry from Stopping You.*

9. ACCOUNTABILITY THROUGH COMMUNITY

i. Power, "Accountability Groups: The Support You Need to Succeed in 2023."

ii. Spina Horan, "10 Signs of a Problem with Perfectionism."

10. FINDING A LIFE WHERE YOU ARE FREE TO BE... JUST BE

i. UCLA, "Understand the body's response to fear & anxiety."
ii. Cleveland Clinic, "How To Heal Your Inner Child."
iii. Friedman, "Women Get Less Exercise Than Men. It's a Problem."
iv. American Society for Nutrition, "What you eat at age 40 could influence your quality of life at age 70."

ABOUT THE AUTHOR

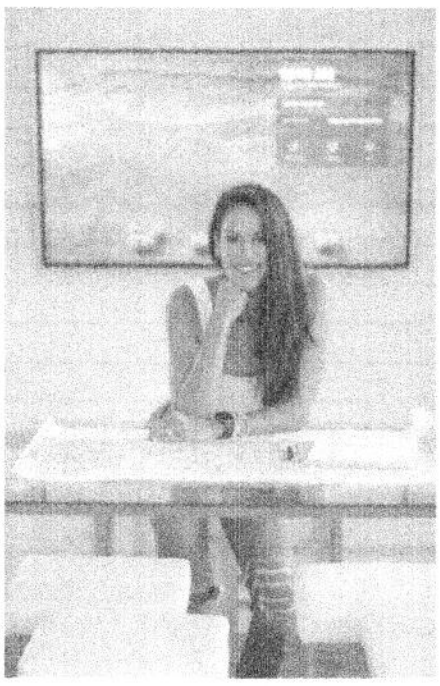

Emily Wright Mitchell is a Texas-raised mother and wife who spreads her passion for health and fitness to women in her community and online. An expert in health and nutrition as a nutritional therapy practitioner, Mitchell's passion comes from years of struggles with both weight and mental health issues.

Today, Mitchell uses both her personal experience and her professional knowledge to guide women in becoming the best version of themselves, teaching them to understand the foundations of health and take back their lives. *Better Than Before* is her first book.

To get Emily's 7-day reset, go to www.betterthanemily.com/reset
or scan the QR code below

ABOUT THE PUBLISHER

LEGACY launch pad PUBLISHING

Legacy Launch Pad is a boutique publishing company that works with entrepreneurs from all over the world.

For more information about Legacy Launch Pad Publishing, go to: www.legacylaunchpadpub.com.

Made in the USA
Monee, IL
05 July 2025

20509132R00100